NUCLEAR MEDICINE

POLICY

&

PROCEDURES*

FOR
NUCLEAR CARDIOLOGY*

By:
Janet Goodrich
John W. McMorris SR CNMT, ASCP (NM)

*Treatment decisions and other medical decisions should be made only by qualified medical personnel in consultation with their patients and should be based, in whole or part, upon the decisions of licensed Physician.

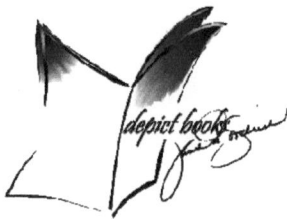

ISBN-10:0990003736
ISBN-13:978-0-9900037-3-1

Published by depict books.
depict books and associated logos are trademarks of depict books.

Nuclear Medicine Manual on CD–includes printable manual, forms and protocols

Contact: editor@depictbooks.com
              depict books
              13714 Briarlake Ave
              Baton Rouge, LA 70809

TABLE OF CONTENTS

In Memory

of

John W. McMorris SR CNMT, ASCP (NM)

1942-2013

PART A   STRUCTURE AND ORGANIZATION

MEMORANDUM

Subject: ***Nuclear Medicine Policy and Procedure Manual***

Annual Policy and Procedure Manual Review Memorandum
(Complete section A or B)

DATE:_____

TO: _____

FROM: _____
                              MEDICAL DIRECTOR

COPY: _____

A
I have performed a review of the ***Nuclear Medicine Policy and Procedure Manual*** and find it to be accurate and complete *(minimum every 3 years).*

_____
MEDICAL DIRECTOR

B
I have performed a review of the ***Nuclear Medicine Policy and Procedure Manual*** and am instituting the following changes *(minimum every 3 years)*:

_____

_____

_____

_____
MEDICAL DIRECTOR

NOTES

SECTION A1.   PERSONNEL AND SUPERVISION

ADMINISTRATOR			
TELEPHONE	FAX	E-MAIL	PAGER/CELL
MEDICAL DIRECTOR			
TELEPHONE	FAX	E-MAIL	PAGER/CELL
RADIATION SAFETY OFFICER			
TELEPHONE	FAX	E-MAIL	PAGER/CELL
TECHNICAL DIRECTOR			
TELEPHONE	FAX	E-MAIL	PAGER/CELL

MEDICAL DIRECTOR		RAM AUTHORIZED USER
		YES NO DATE CERTIFIED

BOARD CERTIFIED PHYSICIAN WITHIN THE PRACTICE	SPECIALTY	RAM AUTHORIZED USER
		YES NO
		DATE CERTIFIED
		YES NO
		DATE CERTIFIED
		YES NO
		DATE CERTIFIED
		YES NO
		DATE CERTIFIED

OTHER PHYSICIANS WHO PRACTICE WITHIN YOUR ENTITY	SPECIALTY	RAM AUTHORIZED USER
		YES NO
		DATE CERTIFIED
OTHER PHYSICIANS WHO PRACTICE WITHIN YOUR ENTITY	SPECIALTY	RAM AUTHORIZED USER

TECHNICAL DIRECTOR					
RT (N)	CNMT	NCT	OTHER	LICENSE NO.	STATE
TELEPHONE	FAX			E-MAIL	PAGEr/CELL

QUALIFICATIONS OF PERSON(S) PERFORMING PROCEDURES

TECHNOLOGIST					
RT (N)	CNMT	NCT	OTHER	LICENSE NO.	*STATE*
TELEPHONE		FAX		E-MAIL	PAGEr/CELL
TECHNOLOGIST					
RT (N)	CNMT	NCT	OTHER	LICENSE NO.	*STATE*
TELEPHONE		FAX		E-MAIL	PAGEr/CELL
TECHNOLOGIST					
RT (N)	CNMT	NCT	OTHER	LICENSE NO.	*STATE*
TELEPHONE		FAX		E-MAIL	PAGEr/CELL
TECHNOLOGIST					
RT (N)	CNMT	NCT	OTHER	LICENSE NO.	*STATE*
TELEPHONE		FAX		E-MAIL	PAGEr/CELL

SECTION A2.   ANCILLARY PERSONNEL

NAME	POSITION	LICENSE OR CERTIFICATIONS	
TELEPHONE	FAX	E-MAIL	PAGER/CELL
TELEPHONE	FAX	E-MAIL	PAGER/CELL
TELEPHONE	FAX	E-MAIL	PAGER/CELL
DATA BACKUP SYSTEM	TYPE	OFF SITE	ONSITE

SECTION A3.   PHYSICAL FACILITIES

GROUP OR PRACTICE NAME	
SPECIALTY	
STREET ADDRESS	
CITY, STATE, ZIP,	
TELEPHONE	FAX		
Website	
ICANL ACCREDITATION DATE	

INSERT FACILITY LICENSE
        RADIOACTIVE MATERIAL LICENSE
        CURRENT NUCLEAR REGULATORY
        RADIOACTIVE MATERIAL INSPECTION

NOTES

INSERT CREDENTIALS
PHYSICIAN CREDENTIALS
PHYSICIAN CV
PHYSICIAN CME

NOTES

INSERT LICENSE
TECHNOLOGISTS CREDENTIALS
TECHNOLOGIST CEU
PERSONNEL LICENSURE
PERSONNEL ACLS/BLS
NURSE CREDENTIALS
NURSE CEU

NOTES

NUCLEAR MEDICINE

SECTION A4. EQUIPMENT AND INSTRUMENTATION

A4.1 Electrical Equipment Safety Policy

PURPOSE:

Policy for and procedure for electrical equipment safety.

Electrical equipment will be inspected and receive preventive maintenance as the manufacturer recommendations suggests and include:

PROCEDURE

1. Bi-annually
   1.1. Inspect treadmills,
   1.2. EKG gate for camera
2. Annually
   2.1. Inspect infusion pumps (battery-operated BAXA is exempt)
   2.2. Plus all other electrical equipment that touches the patient.
3. Ensure that all electrical machinery to be plugged in outlets are approved for the particular device.
4. If equipment exhibits an electrical problem, the unit should be unplugged and manufacturer or maintenance notified
5. Defibrillators must be checked daily to ensure working capability according to manufacturer's instruction.
6. Monthly
   6.1. Radiation monitoring devices
   6.2. Resuscitation equipment
7. If applicable
   7.1. Hood for volatile radionuclide or cell handling
   7.2. Xenon (or other gas) trap

NOTES

NUCLEAR MEDICINE
SECTION A4.2   EQUIPMENT AND INSTRUMENTATION IN USE

EQUIPMENT AND INSTRUMENTATION IN USE

TYPE	MANUFACTURER	MODEL	YEAR
Dose calibrator or decay correction calculation system			
Imaging/counting (i.e. gamma camera, uptake probe, etc)			
Radiation safety monitoring devices (portable survey meter)			
Removable contamination equipment or well counter			
Resuscitation equipment (AED or suction etc)			
Exercise equipment (i.e. treadmill or bicycle)			
Exercise equipment (i.e. treadmill or bicycle)			
ECG equipment (stress testing and ECG gate)			
ECG equipment (stress testing and ECG gate)			
Ancillary monitoring equipment (i.e. pulse oximeter)			
Infusion pumps/automated injectors			
Glucometer			
Fume hood			
Xenon gas and dispensing and delivery system			
Medication refrigerators			
Dose management system			

Accepted by: _____ (Initials) Date_____   .

NOTES

NUCLEAR MEDICINE
SECTION A5   VOLUME OF CLINICAL PROCEDURES

PROCEDURE:

The annual procedure volume is sufficient to maintain proficiency in examination interpretation and performance. It is recommended that a facility should perform a minimum of 600 Nuclear Medicine Patient Procedures Annually.

The initial requirement before a laboratory may apply for accreditation is six months in existence and a minimum of 300 Nuclear Cardiology and/or 600 general Nuclear Medicine procedures. This number is based on the importance of performing a sufficient number of studies to determine and maintain proficiency. Therefore, annual volume is sufficient if it follows the ICANL recommendation - 300/Yr Nuclear Cardiology; 600/Yr General Nuclear

ICANL does not have a set standard for the number of studies to be read by each cardiologist per year, however, we highly recommend that the annual procedure volume be sufficient to maintain proficiency in exam interpretation and performance.

Volume of Examinations_____

NOTES

PART B   PROCEDURES AND PROTOCOLS

B1.1.4   Employee Orientation-Annual Checklist*

PURPOSE: New employee review orientation and standards to set annual due date coinciding with hire date or facility policy date. Employees with access to Ram to be reviewed annually by supervisor

	EMPLOYEE: _____	DATE: _____
	EMERGENCY CONTACT NUMBER: _____	Page ___ of ___
	EMPLOYEE ORIENTATION AND ANNUAL CHECKLIST	
☐	Assignment of locker / Department keys	
☐	Location of Emergency Equipment/O2 Tanks	
☐	R.A.C.E.	
☐	P.A.S.S.	
☐	Patient Preparation for Exams	
☐	Patient Identification/CCSS requests	
☐	Procedure for Nuclear Exams on Pregnant/ Lactating Patients	
☐	Radionuclide Dosages for Each Exam/ Pediatric Dosing	
☐	Injection Techniques/Y Connectors	
☐	Misadministration (Medical Events)	
☐	Scheduling Guidelines MPI/ One Day/Two Day	
☐	Scheduling Guidelines for Adenosine / Dobutamine/_____	
☐	Film and Image Labeling / Archiving studies	
☐	Wet Book Recording / Setting up Evening Conference	
☐	Review of ongoing Research Protocols	
☐	Ultra Tag kit Preparation/ In Vivo Tagging	
☐	Radiopharmacy Manuals	
☐	Equipment QC / Service Calls	
☐	Universal Precautions / Personal Safety / Body Mechanics	
☐	Treadmill	
	HOTLAB CHECKLIST	
☐	Package Surveys / Wipe test/ Log book	
☐	Dose Labels	
☐	Aseptic technique	
☐	Assay in Dose Calibrator/ Radiopharmaceutical log sheets Syntrac system *(If applicable)*	
☐	Dose calibrator QC	
☐	Daily Surveys	
☐	Hot Trash/Separating sharps	
☐	Label and log in trash to be stored/Bins for storage downstairs	
☐	Surveys of trash and decay room	

EMPLOYEE: _____ **DATE:** _____

EMERGENCY CONTACT NUMBER: _____ **Page** ___ **of** ___

☐	Label and log in trash to be stored/Bins for storage downstairs	
☐	Rotation schedules /tardiness / overtime / time card	
☐	PTO: scheduled, unscheduled, holidays	
☐	On-call policy	
	Radiation Safety / ALARA / Personal Monitoring	
☐	Technologist Pregnancy Policy	
☐	Criteria Based Performance Reviews	
☐	Attendance at Staff Meetings and In service Education Seminars	
☐	Radiation Spills / Radiation Accident Plan	
☐	Diagnostic Imaging Disaster Plan	
☐	**COPY OF POLICIES**	
☐	Mission Statement	
☐	Employee conduct and Discipline	
☐	Service Standards	
☐	Attendance Policy, Vacation Policy	
☐	Dress Code	
☐	Patient Identification, Patient Assessment	
☐	Handling of Non-Radioactive Pharmaceuticals	
☐	Pharmaceuticals are properly stored	
☐	Pharmaceuticals are properly prepared	
☐	All staff is competent in the care of patients with vision impairments.	
☐	All staff is trained for handling special medical needs such as IV's, wounds, catheters, and Oxygen tanks and tubing.	
☐	Patients confined to a wheelchair or cart will be lifted using a draw-sheet technique.	
☐	If a patient becomes violent, threatening, or combative, the supervising physician will be notified, as will the facility security department if necessary.	
☐		
☐		
☐		

SEE ALSO *B4.3.1.4 Radiation Safety Personnel Hire/Annual Review

_____ has reviewed all of the above policies and procedures for Nuclear Medicine with the orienting technologist and/or coordinator.

_____Employee Signature / Date

_____Supervisor Signature / Date
Accepted by: _____ (Initials) Date_____

NUCLEAR MEDICINE

    B2.1   Facility Clinical Procedure Guideline/Form

PURPOSE:

ALL PROCEDURES EXCEPT IMAGING

PROCEDURE TITLE:	
Describe in detail *(Tab to next line)*	
1. *EXPLAIN PURPOSE OF TASK*	
2. *GIVE SPECIFIC STEPS TO ACCOMPLISH TASK – 1, 2, 3, 4, 5 ETC*	
3. *EXPLAIN OUTCOME EXPECTED*	
4. *EXPLAIN EMPLOYEE'S ROLE*	

Accepted by: _____ (Initials) Date_____

NOTES

NUCLEAR MEDICINE
B2.1.1   Patient Identification Process

PURPOSE:

To establish guidelines for patient identification.

PROCEDURE:

Patient Identification:
1. Patient will check in at the front desk and the clerk will notify the Nuclear Medicine Department.
2. The Nuclear Technologist will confirm patient identity and verify appropriateness of exam according to the written order.
3. Prior to radiopharmaceutical administration, the patient's identity will be verified by more than one method to identify the individual named on the written directive or order.
4. Check patient's license or other personal identification and compare to records.
5. The person performing the procedure will ask
    - ☐ Patient's name
    - ☐ Date of birth or social security number,
    - ☐ Verify information in the patient's record or requisition.
6. Each radiopharmaceutical administration will be in accordance with the ordered procedure and any deviation from the ordered procedure, intended or otherwise, will be identified, evaluated, and appropriate action will be taken.

Accepted by: _____ (Initials) Date_____   .

NOTES

NUCLEAR MEDICINE

B2.1.1   Patient Identification

Welcome to our practice.
Please complete the following form as completely as possible to establish your patient record.
Thank You.

Patient Name _____

Address: _____

City: _____ State: _____ Zip: _____

Home Phone: _____ Work Phone: _____ Cell Phone: _____

Date of Birth: _____ Sex: _____ Married: _____ Single: _____

Social Security Number_____ Employer: _____

Primary Care Physician: _____Referring Physician: _____

Insurance Information
Name of insured: _____

Relationship to Patient: ☐Self Spouse ☐Parent or Legal Guardian (*please check one*)

Insurance Company Name: _____

Policy Number: _____

Insured's Address:
City: _____ State: _____ Zip: _____

Home Phone: _____ Work Phone: _____ Cell Phone: _____

Social Security Number_____ Employer: _____

Allergies: _____

_____
We only discuss medical or billing information with your permission. Please indicate to whom, other than you, we are allowed to release or discuss information, their relationship to you and what information we may disclose.

MEDICAL / BILLING (Please Circle)

Name _____ Relationship to Patient _____

MEDICAL / BILLING (Please Circle)

Name _____ Relationship to Patient _____

Patient's signature or legal guardian: _____

SIGNED _____ DATE_____
                    Accepted by: _____ *(Initials) Date*_____   .

NOTES

NUCLEAR MEDICINE

B2.1.2   Pregnancy/Breastfeeding Screening Protocol

PURPOSE:

To establish guidelines for assessment of female patients.

∴ Signs are posted within the department and waiting areas that state: "If you think you may be pregnant or are breastfeeding, please notify the technologist before your exam".

∴ The technologist must ask all female patients age 12 or older if they are or may be pregnant and if they are breastfeeding an infant/child.

PROCEDURE:

1. The following must be completed prior to starting an exam:
2. Patient must be properly identified and the written order is verified for appropriateness.
3. The general condition and stability of the patient is clinically assessed.
4. The pregnant or potentially pregnant patient is not to have Nuclear Medicine procedures performed unless it is essential for a diagnosis or treatment
5. If the patient appears uncomfortable or unstable, the cardiologist will evaluate the patient.
6. All female patients between the ages of 11 and 60 are asked if there is any chance of pregnancy or if breastfeeding and this is documented on the *Patient Consent Form.*
7. Or Nuclear Medicine testing will not be performed until the patient receives lab work via urine pregnancy test or serum blood test (per physician discretion) declaring no chance of pregnancy.
8. The referring physician may be contacted if there is a chance of pregnancy or breastfeeding as to whether scanning procedures are still needed.
9. If the patient is breastfeeding, the Radiation Safety Officer, or the Health Physics Consultant will be notified before the Nuclear Medicine procedure is performed and the "Breastfeeding Instructions" sheet will be completed and given to the patient.
10. Per the referring or supervising physician, if the benefit of the diagnostic information outweighs the risk of radiation exposure, the technologist will continue with the procedure.
11. When Nuclear Medicine procedures are performed on patients who are breastfeeding, patients must be counseled before administration of the radiopharmaceutical; and must agree to discontinue breastfeeding during specified time.
12. If it is decided by the above that the Nuclear Medicine procedure is necessary, the patient must agree to discontinue breastfeeding for the period prescribed by the Authorized User, Radiation Safety Officer, or Health Physicist.
13. Written instructions regarding the length of time to discontinue nursing must be signed by the patient before the dose is administered and documented in the
14. The patient must sign a consent form before the procedure can be started.
15. Patient will be given a copy of a completed "Instructions for Breastfeeding Patients" form.
16. Original consent form is to be maintained in the patient's chart.
17. If the patient is neither post-menopausal nor surgically sterile and whose last menstrual period began within the past 10 days, the technologist must consult with the Authorized User before administering the radiopharmaceutical dose.
18. See the Table "Recommended Breastfeeding Interruption Times"

Accepted by: _____ (Initials) Date_____   .

NUCLEAR MEDICINE

      B2.1.2   Pregnancy/Breastfeeding Screening Questionnaire

      B2.1.4   Breastfeeding Screening Protocol

TO BE COMPLETED BY ALL FEMALE PATIENTS

Patient's Name _____ Patient ID# _____

Are you (check the appropriate box):

☐ Post-menopausal

☐ Pre-menopausal, surgically sterile (e.g. hysterectomy, tubal ligation)

☐ Pre-menopausal, not surgically sterile.

☐ Are you or do you think you may be pregnant.   ☐Yes ☐No

1. Are you currently breastfeeding: ☐Yes ☐No

2. Date of your last menstrual period: _____

3. Have you ever had a mastectomy   ☐Yes ☐No

                                   ☐ Right

              ☐   Left

              Implant/Prosthesis   ☐ Right

              Implant/Prosthesis   ☐ Left

Patient's Signature: _____ Date: _____

Accepted by: _____ (Initials) Date_____ .

NUCLEAR MEDICINE
B2.1.2.3   Fetal Exposure Protocol

PURPOSE:
To establish a procedure for fetal radiation exposure from diagnostic Nuclear Medicine procedures.

PROCEDURE:
The radiation associated with diagnostic Nuclear Medicine procedures is similar to that of other diagnostic procedures such as X-rays. There is a difference, however, between how X-rays are transmitted through the region imaged – chest, abdomen, pelvis, and bone, and administration of orally or intravenously radioactive material, which generally localizes primarily in one part or organ of the body, e. g. lung scan, thyroid scan.

Potential Fetal Exposure:
1. Women of childbearing age who could be pregnant at the time of Nuclear Medicine procedures will be questioned about their last menstrual period and may need to undergo a pregnancy test before proceeding.
2. The pregnant or potentially pregnant patient is not to have a Nuclear Medicine procedure in this lab unless the benefits of the procedures diagnostic information will outweigh the radiation risk to the embryo/fetus.
3. Before any diagnostic test, patients are requested to tell the technologist if they may be pregnant.
4. The consequences of radiation exposure to a fetus or embryo from a diagnostic Nuclear Medicine test are usually insignificant. Nonetheless, if the diagnostic test is an elective procedure as opposed to an urgent or life-threatening procedure, it can be postponed and rescheduled until a negative pregnancy test can be obtained.
5. Signs must be prominently displayed in the department the pregnancy exposure policy.
6. If a patient is pregnant, the Authorized User must be informed and the necessity of the procedure discussed. Alternative procedures should be considered, such as ultrasound, to determine if adequate diagnostic information could be determined from methods other than the Nuclear Medicine study.

Fetal Radiation Dose Calculations:
1. Patients who are pregnant and receive a radioactive dose intended or unintended, must have the fetal dose determined. The determination of the dose to the embryo/fetus from the intake of radioactive material by the pregnant woman should be based on the best available scientific information. This dose is to be determined by the Authorized User, Radiation Safety Officer, and or Health Physicist. The method to determine the dose should be based upon *Revision 1 to NUREG/CR-5631*.

2. The referring physician must be contacted prior to the procedure. Upon discussion with the Authorized User, Radiation Safety Officer and or the Health Physicists, the referring physician should decide whether the procedure is clinical indicated, and the benefits of the procedure will out weigh the risk to the embryo/fetus. The pregnant patient should be informed of the risks to the embryo/fetus by the injection or ingestion of the radioactive material. An informed consent should be made.

3. If a patient receives a radioactive dose while pregnant unintentionally, upon learning of the pregnancy, the lab will determine the dose to the embryo/fetus. This dose is to be determined by the Authorized User, Radiation Safety Officer, and or a Health Physicist.

4. The method to determining the dose should be based upon *Revision 1 to NUREG/CR-5631*. The Authorized User, Radiation Safety Officer, and or Health Physicists will then discuss the information on the dose to embryo/fetus with the referring physician and the patient.

PROCEDURE:

1. Calculating the fetal dose to a pregnant patient receiving a radiopharmaceutical for clinical Nuclear Medicine procedures is based on the method of Russell and Stabin, "Radiation Absorbed Dose to the Embryo/Fetus from Radiopharmaceuticals", Health Physics, November 1997. (See Section B4 TABLES A,B,C)

2. The fetal dose is estimated from tables of radiopharmaceuticals listing the fetal dose based on the amount of radiopharmaceutical administered to the patient–e.g. the fetal dose from a pregnant patient administered 30mCi of Tc-99m Sestamibi is 1.3rad.

3. Tables A,B, C from this reference are used. The fetal dose can be from maternal and fetal self dose contributions. The more extensive data is listed for maternal contributions only. Some radiopharmaceuticals are not found in the Stabin article–e.g. Tc99m Myoview (Tetrofosmin).

4. In such cases International Council on Radiation Protection Report No. 53 (ICRP 53) can be used to approximate the fetal dose from the dose to the uterus. ICRP 53 contains tables for most radiopharmaceuticals. With the tables complete, most dose calculations are just a matter of lookup and perhaps interpolation.

5. Given the uncertainties in the numbers, careful interpolation may not be needed. In most cases, one can look at the dose on either side of the actual time of gestation, and just use what is felt to be the most appropriate, most conservative, estimate. During the first, say, 3-6 weeks, the dose to the nongravid uterus (the "early pregnancy" dose) is probably a good estimate of the dose to the fetus.

    5.1. Example - A woman receives 1000 MBq of Tc-99m MIBI for a cardiac stress test. Later it is found out that she was about 1 week pregnant at the time of the scan. Here, the most appropriate fetal dose is 1000 MBq x 0.012 mGy/MBq = 12 mGy.

    5.2. Example - A woman receives 200 MBq of Tc-99m MAA for a lung scan at about 7 months' gestation (this is not unusual - some women have a tendency to form blood clots in later pregnancy, and lung scans are often performed on patients known to be pregnant). The dose estimate at 6 months is 200 MBq x 0.005 mGy/MBq = 1 mGy, and the estimate at 9 months is 200 MBq x 0.004 mGy/MBq = 0.8 mGy. Given the uncertainty and the time, I would call the dose estimate 1 mGy.

NUCLEAR MEDICINE
B2.1.2.3   Fetal Exposure Record

Licensee: _____

Address: _____

City: _____ State: _____, Zip: _____

This report calculates the fetal dose to _____, the

patient that was approximately _____ weeks pregnant.

The patient received

_____mCi of Tc-99m for a rest cardiac study and

_____ mCi of Tc-99m _____ for a stress

cardiac study on _____

∴   The absorbed dose to the embryo/fetus per unit activity administered to the mother (maternal

   contributions only) in early pregnancy:

Tc-99m MIBI rest: 0.015 mGy/MBq

Tc-99m MIBI stress: 0.012 mGy/MBq

[from Russel, Stabin, Spraks, Watson, "Radiation Absorbed Dose to the Embryo/Fetus from
Radiopharmaceuticals," Health Physics, November 1997, Volume 73, Number 5]

∴   Calculation of fetal dose based on administered activity to the mother (from maternal dose

   contributions):

0.015mGy/MBq   x37MBq/mCi x_____mCi x 100mrad/mGy =_____ mrad

0.012mGy/MBq   x37MBq/mCi x_____mCi x 100mrad/mGy =_____ mrad

The total fetal dose is _____mrad or _____rad.

This is well below the 5 rad that the National Council on Radiation Protection considers as a

negligible risk when compared to other risks of pregnancy.

Accepted by: _____ (Initials) Date_____   .

NUCLEAR MEDICINE
> B2.1.2.4   Unintended Radiation Exposure to Fetus

PURPOSE:
Reporting unintended radiation exposure greater than 5 rem to fetus or nursing child.

PROCEDURE:
Reports of Exposures, Radiation Levels, and Concentrations of Radioactive Material Exceeding the Constraints or Limits
1. Reportable Events. In addition to the notification required, each licensee or registrant shall submit a written report to the Office of Environmental Compliance using the procedures provided and within 30 days after learning of any of the following occurrences:
2. Incidents for which notification is required
3. Doses in excess of any of the following:
    - 3.1.   the occupational dose limits for adults
    - 3.2.   the occupational dose limits for a minor
    - 3.3.   the limits for an embryo/fetus of a declared pregnant woman
    - 3.4.   the limits for an individual member of the public
    - 3.5.   any applicable limit in the license or registration; or
    - 3.6.   the ALARA constraints for air emissions established
4. Levels of radiation or concentrations of radioactive material in:
    - 4.1.   a restricted area in excess of applicable limits in license or registration; or
    - 4.2.   an unrestricted area in excess of 10 times the applicable limit set forth in this
    Chapter or in the license or registration, whether or not involving exposure of any individual in excess of the limits or
5. For licensees subject to the provisions of U.S. Environmental protection agency's generally applicable environmental radiation standards in 40 CFR Part 190, levels of radiation or releases of radioactive material in excess of those standards, or of license conditions related to those standards.

CONTENTS OF REPORTS
1. Each report required shall describe the extent of exposure of individuals to radiation and radioactive material, including, as appropriate:
    - 1.1.   estimates of each individual's dose;
    - 1.2.   the levels of radiation and concentrations of radioactive material involved;
    - 1.3.   the cause of the elevated exposures, dose rates, or concentrations;
    - 1.4.   corrective steps taken or planned to ensure against a recurrence, including the schedule for achieving conformance with applicable limits, ALARA constraints, generally applicable environmental standards, and associated license or registration conditions; and
    - 1.5.   information required if the overexposure involves failure of safety components of radiography equipment.

1.6.   Each report filed in accordance with Subsection A of this Section shall include for each occupationally overexposed individual the name, driver's license or state identification number and the issuing state, and date of birth. With respect to the limit for the embryo/fetus the identifiers should be those of the declared pregnant woman. The report shall be prepared so that this information is stated in a separate and detachable portion of the report.

All licensees or registrants who make reports shall submit the report in writing to the department

of: (Required Regulatory Agency)_____.

REPORTS OF PLANNED SPECIAL EXPOSURES

∴   The licensee or registrant shall submit a written report within 30 days following any planned special exposure informing _____ that a planned special exposure was conducted and indicating the date the planned special exposure occurred and the information required.

REPORTS OF INDIVIDUAL MONITORING

This Section applies to each person licensed or registered by the department to:
1. Possess or use sources of radiation for purposes of industrial radiography
2. Receive radioactive waste from other persons for disposal or
3. Possess or use at any time, for purposes of processing or manufacturing for distribution radioactive material in quantities exceeding any one of the following quantities:

Radionuclide	Activity a	
	Ci	GBq
Cesium-137	1	37
Cobalt-60	1	37
Gold-198	100	3,700
Iodine-131	1	37
Iridium-192	10	370
Krypton-85	1,000	37,000
Promethium-147	10	370
Technetium-99m	1,000	37,000

4. The department may require as a license condition, or by rule or regulation, reports from licensees or registrants who are licensed or registered to use radionuclides not on this list, in quantities sufficient to cause comparable radiation levels.

5. Each licensee or registrant in a category listed in Subsection A of this Section shall submit to the Office of Environmental Compliance, an annual report of the results of individual monitoring carried out by the licensee or

6. registrant for each individual for whom monitoring was required during that year. The licensee or registrant may include additional data for individuals for whom monitoring was provided but not required.

7. The licensee or registrant shall file the report required by Subsection B of this Section, covering the preceding year, on or before _____ of each year. The licensee or registrant shall submit the report to the Office of Environmental Compliance,

_____

NUCLEAR MEDICINE
B2.1.3 Recommended Breastfeeding Interruption Times
PROCEDURE:
Table 3 (See Also: Journal of Nuclear Medicine, Volume 41, pages 863-873, 2000).
Summary of Recommendations for Radiopharmaceuticals Excreted in the Breast Milk

Pharmaceutical	Activity, mCi (MBq)	Counseling ?*	Advisory		
Ga-67 Citrate	5.0 (185)	Yes	Cessation		
Tc-99m DTPA	20 (740)	No			
Tc-99m MAA	4 (148)	Yes	12 hr		
Tc-99m Pertechnetate	5 (185)	Yes	4 hr		
I-131 NaI	150 (5550)	Yes	Cessation		
Cr-51 EDTA	0.05 (1.85)	No			
Tc-99m DISIDA	8 (300)	No			
Tc-99m glucoheptonate	20 (740)	No			
Tc-99m HAM	8 (300)	No			
Tc-99m MIBI		30 (1110)	No		
Tc-99m MDP	20 (740)	No			
Tc-99m PYP	20 (740)	No			
Tc-99m RBC's in vivo	20 (740)	Yes	12 hr		
Tc-99m RBC's in vitro	20(740)	No			
Tc-99m Sulfur Colloid	12 (444)	No			
In-111 WBC's	0.5 (18.5)	No			
I-123 NaI	0.4 (14.8)	Yes	Cessation		
I-123 OIH	2 (74)	No			
I-123 MIBG	10 (370)	Yes	48 hr		
I-125 OIH	0.01 (0.37)	No			
I-131 OIH	0.3 (11.1)	No			
Tc-99m DTPA Aerosol	1 (37)	No			
Tc-99m MAG3	10 (370)	No			
Tc-99m WBC's	5 (185)	Yes	48 hr		
Tl-201	3 (111)	Yes	96 hr		

* *"No" means that interruption of breast feeding need not be suggested, given the criterion of a limit of 1 mSv ED to the infant and these amounts of administered activity.*

* *"Yes" means that some interruption is required, as noted in the next column.*

As noted in Rev. 1 to NUREG/CR-5631, ICRP Publication 30 (Ref. C2) employs a metabolic model in which a fraction of activity in the first transfer compartment (blood) often is assumed to go immediately to excretion. Because of the minuscule mass of the embryo/fetus immediately following fertilization, for some materials the biokinetic model thus predicts that there would be negligible initial activity in the embryo after administration at that time, and that there would be minimal activity at later times. As a consequence, the dose rate and doses also would be negligible, which is indicated by N in the table. For these nuclides, an approximation of the cumulative dose for an intake occurring during the first 30 days should be made based on a time-weighted average of the 31-day intake data. The cumulative dose from an intake in the first 30 days of pregnancy may be estimated by multiplying the 31-day cumulated dose value by the ratio of the days-to-date in the first month to a 30-day period.

For example, assuming a maternal intake of C-14 resulting in a 1 μCi blood uptake on the 20th day of the pregnancy, the gestation dose should be determined by multiplying the cumulative dose from an intake at day 31 (i.e., Table C3, Cumulated Dose column, 1.89E-04 rads) by the ratio of 20 days to 30 days (i.e., 20 divided by 30).

2.3.2 Method Using Revision 1 to NUREG/CR-5631

Using the methods of NUREG/CR-5631, the dose to the embryo/fetus is calculated in a manner similar to that of the Simplified Method,

The first column of Table C1 presents the gestation time (e.g., 0, 30, 60 days), and the last column presents the cumulated dose to the embryo/fetus for the remainder of the gestation period following the introduction of unit activity into maternal blood at the specified gestation time. As specified paragraph 3.2.2, an intake at any time within a specific monthly gestation period (i.e., a 30-day period) may be assumed to have occurred at the beginning of the monthly period for the purpose of determining the appropriate dose factor to be used. For example, for intakes occurring during the first month of pregnancy, the dose factor under the "Cumulated Dose" column corresponding to 0 days of gestation (as designated in the left-most column of the table) should be used. Cumulated dose factors taken from Table C1 for intakes in the respective months of gestation are presented below:

Stage of Gestation at Time of Intake	Cumulated Dose Factor for Remainder of Gestation Period (rad/μCi, blood)
1st Month (0 - 30 days)	9.03E-06
2nd Month (31 - 60 days)	1.77E-05
3rd Month (61 - 90 days)	4.02E-05

Using these gestation-time dependent dose factors, the dose equivalent to the embryo/fetus is calculated using the regulatory position specified in subsection 3.2. The radiation quality factor for H-3 is 1.0. The dose to the embryo/fetus for the remainder of the gestation period resulting from intakes occurring within each month is calculated as follows:

Dose Equivalent = Intake x fl x DFi

First-month intake: 156 μCi x 1.0 x 9.03E-06 rad/μCi x 1.0 rem/rad = 0.001 rem

Second-month intake: 248 μCi x 1.0 x 1.77E-05 rad/μCi x 1.0 rem/rad = 0.004 rem

Third-month intake: 185 μCi x 1.0 x 4.02E-05 rad/μCi x 1.0 rem/rad = 0.007 rem

TOTAL = 0.013 rem*

* The difference between the sum of the monthly doses and the total (i.e., 0.012 rem versus 0.013 rem) is caused by rounding.

In keeping with the recommendation contained in the Discussion section of this guide, final results should be rounded to the nearest thousandth of a rem.

Radiopharmaceutical	Procedure	Dose	Breastfeeding Interruption Time
Tc Labeled RBCs	Gated Heart	30 mCi	9 hours 1
	GI Bleed, Liver, Hemangioma	20 mCi	6 hours 1
Tc MIBI/Myoview	Cardiac Studies	30 mCi	3 hours 2
Tc Pertechnetate	Cardiac shunt, left right shunt	20 mCi	24 hours 1
All others listed on the Dose List			NA 1

[1] *US Nuclear Regulatory Commission, Regulatory Guide 8.39, "Release of Patient's Administered Radioactive Materials", April 1997.*

[2] *US Nuclear Regulatory Commission, NUREG-1492, "Regulatory Analysis of Criteria for the Release of Patients Administered Radioactive Materials", February 1997.*

NUCLEAR MEDICINE
B2.1.3   Pregnancy and Breastfeeding Instruction

Patient Name: _____ Date: _____

     Your physician has referred you to _____ for the following

procedure: _____

     During this procedure, you will be administered a small amount of radioactive material.

     You have also indicated that you are currently breastfeeding an infant/child. Please follow the instructions indicated below relating to breastfeeding after the administration of the radioactive material.

- ☐ Interrupt the breastfeeding for a period of _____
- ☐ Small quantities of the radioactive material you will be administered will be present in your breast milk following the examination. Although failure to interrupt your breastfeeding will not produce any noticeable adverse effects in your infant/child, it is prudent to avoid the unnecessary radiation exposure to your infant/child during the interruption time recommended above. You may continue breastfeeding your infant/child after the interruption recommended period. At that time, your child will not receive any significant radiation exposure because of continuing breastfeeding.

- ☐ No interruption of breastfeeding is necessary.
- ☐ Although you are being administered a radioactive material, the radiation exposure to your infant/child will not be significant, even if breastfeeding is continued.

Patient's Signature _____ Date _____

Witness _____ Date _____

       Accepted by: _____ (Initials) Date_____   .

NUCLEAR MEDICINE
SECTION 2. IMAGING PROCEDURE PROTOCOLS
B2.2   Diagnostic Imaging Procedure Protocol Guideline

PURPOSE:

To evaluate regional myocardial perfusion at rest and under stress (either physical exercise or pharmacologic stress).

To identify and localize areas of reversible ischemia or previous infarction in patients with chest pain, suspected of having coronary artery disease, previous coronary intervention, or previous abnormal ECG examination.

HISTORY:

(e.g. 65-yr woman with known coronary artery disease and recurrent chest pain).

CLINICAL INDICATIONS:

Myocardial perfusion imaging (MPI) is indicated for the detection of coronary artery disease (CAD) and for assessing prognosis in patients with symptoms suggestive of CAD or with risk factors for CAD. Pharmacologic stress MPI is indicated as an adjunct to radionuclide MPI in patients unable to exercise adequately. Physical limitations or circumstances that may prevent patients from exercising adequately include:

- Peripheral vascular disease
- Musculoskeletal and neurological disorders
- Pulmonary disease
- Treatment with medications that blunt heart rate response
- Recent acute myocardial infarction (within 3-5 days)
-

CONTRAINDICATIONS

- Acute MI
- Recent MI
- Unstable angina
- Acute myocarditis or pericarditis
- Heart block greater than first degree (second or third degree heart block0
- PaO2 < 40 mmHg on room air
- Rapid arrythmias
- Orthopedic problems
- CHF (uncompensated)
- Significant aortic stenosis
- HTN (uncontrolled)
- Pulmonary hypertension

PATIENT PREPARATION

1. Patients should be instructed about food or diet restrictions.
2. Add department procedure (NPO or light meal), include number of hours prior to exam
3. Patients should avoid foods containing caffeine for 24 hours prior to the examination. These include:
    3.1. Chocolate and cocoa
    3.2. Coffee and tea to include any decaffeinated brands
    3.3. Colas or soft drinks containing caffeine, including those with "caffeine-free" labels
    3.4. Aspirin containing caffeine
    3.5. Indicate other food or diet restrictions as appropriate

4. In consultation with the referring physician, consider discontinuation of specific medications prior to the procedure. Depending on the indication for stress testing and the clinical question to be answered, it may be advisable to discontinue certain medications. e.g. Calcium Channel Blockers and Beta Blocking Drugs
    4.1. _____
    4.2. _____
5. Patients should be instructed about withholding medications.
6. Include patient instruction sheet

PATIENT PREPARATION – DAY OF TEST

1. Explain the procedure and possible side effects of the pharmacologic stress agent.
2. Assess for pregnancy and breastfeeding.
3. Obtain a signed consent form.
4. Add other patient preparations as appropriate

ADMINISTERED ACTIVITY

1. Technetium-99m Sestamibi
2. Product name administered via intravenous injection:
3. Rest: [value] 10mCi
4. Stress: [value]30mCi

ADENOSINE STRESS PATIENTS ONLY:

1. Non-radioactive drugs—Aminophylline:
2. Dose: [value] 125 mg
3. Intravenous infusion
4. Timing of administration: [value] If needed wait 2 minutes after injection to give Aminophylline
5. Precautions/Restrictions: [value] Do not give to patients allergic to Xanthines

CAMERA MAKE MODEL:

INCLUDE:

1. Emergency Procedures
    1.1. Emergency Shutdown
    1.2. Location of Emergency Buttons, Controls, Electrical
2. Describe System Power-up and Logon Procedure
    2.1. Be specific e.g. Press Red Button in lower left corner
3. Describe in detail camera quality control procedure and frequency
4. Explain how to access data and purpose
5. Explain purpose of imaging procedure
6. Tell how to setup camera in detail including 1-6 below
7. Describe Processing Data
    7.1. Be Specific e. g.
        7.1.1. Prefilters, filter cutoff/power, motion correction, reconstruction filter
8. Describe Image Filming
9. Listing for camera manufacturer Help-Line
10. Add as many pages and details as needed to operate equipment.

Camera setup (collimator, energy window setting, etc)

Patient and camera positioning

Camera/computer specific acquisition protocols including timing of views, time/counts per view, number of views as well as specific parameters and filtering including orbit, number of stops, time per stop, ECG-gating set-up

Camera/computer specific processing and reconstruction protocols, including standards for filtering

Camera/computer specific display protocols

Appropriate image labeling including name, patient identification, date and type of study, time interval as appropriate, view or projection and anatomical markers as appropriate

**Typist: Please have Nuclear Tech review Protocol before entering in manual

PROCEDURE:	
Describe in detail (Tab to next line)	

1. *EXPLAIN PURPOSE OF TASK*
2. *GIVE SPECIFIC STEPS TO ACCOMPLISH TASK – 1, 2, 3, 4, 5 ETC*
3. *EXPLAIN OUTCOME EXPECTED*
4. *EXPLAIN EMPLOYEE'S ROLE*

NUCLEAR MEDICINE
>B2.2   Diagnostic Imaging Procedure Protocols
>Myocardial Perfusion Imaging Same-Day Rest/Stress Tc99m
>*Two-Day Stress/Rest Tc99m

PURPOSE:

To evaluate regional myocardial perfusion at rest and under stress (either physical exercise or pharmacologic stress).

To identify and localize areas of reversible ischemia or previous infarction in patients with chest pain, suspected of having coronary artery disease, previous coronary intervention, or previous abnormal ECG examination.

Add others as appropriate

HISTORY:

(e.g. 65-yr woman with known coronary artery disease and recurrent chest pain).

CLINICAL INDICATIONS:

Myocardial perfusion imaging (MPI) is indicated for the detection of coronary artery disease (CAD) and for assessing prognosis in patients with symptoms suggestive of CAD or with risk factors for CAD. Pharmacologic stress MPI is indicated as an adjunct to radionuclide MPI in patients unable to exercise adequately. Physical limitations or circumstances that may prevent patients from exercising adequately include:

- ☐ Peripheral vascular disease
- ☐ Musculoskeletal and neurological disorders
- ☐ Pulmonary disease
- ☐ Treatment with medications that blunt heart rate response
- ☐ Recent acute myocardial infarction (within 3-5 days)
- ☐ List others as appropriate

CONTRAINDICATIONS

List as appropriate

- ☐ Chest pain consistent with unstable angina.
- ☐ Back or leg injuries or severe handicap that precludes use of the treadmill.
- ☐ Decompensated or inadequately controlled CHF.
- ☐ Uncontrolled blood pressure (e.g. resting BP >200/115 mmHg).
- ☐ Acute or recent myocardial infarction within last 2-3 days.
- ☐ Uncontrolled cardiac arrhythmias.
- ☐ Rapid arrhythmias

- ☐ Acute PE.
- ☐ Unwillingness to give consent.
- ☐ Acute myocarditis, endocarditis, pericarditis.
- ☐ Significant or Severe aortic stenosis.
- ☐ Hypertrophic obstructive cardiomyopathy.
- ☐ Patients with LBBB or A-V paced rhythm.
- ☐ Unstable angina
- ☐ Heart block greater than first degree (second or third degree heart block0
- ☐ PaO2 < 40 mmHg on room air
- ☐ Orthopedic problems
- ☐ CHF (uncompensated)
- ☐ Pulmonary hypertension

PATIENT EDUCATION/INSTRUCTIONS
Patients should be instructed about any food or diet restrictions.
Add department procedure (NPO or light meal) including number of hours prior to exam

_____

_____

_____

Patients should avoid foods containing caffeine for 24 hours prior to the examination. These include:
- ☐ Chocolate and cocoa
- ☐ Coffee and tea to include any decaffeinated brands
- ☐ Colas or any soft drinks containing caffeine, including those with "caffeine-free" labels
- ☐ Aspirin containing caffeine
- ☐ Indicate other food or diet restrictions as appropriate

_____

_____

In consultation with the referring physician, consider discontinuation of specific medications prior to the procedure. Depending on the indication for stress testing and the clinical question to be answered, it may be advisable to discontinue certain medications.
- ☐ Patients should be instructed about withholding medications.
- ☐ Include patient instruction sheet

PATIENT PREPARATION – DAY OF TEST
- ☐ Explain the procedure and possible side effects of the pharmacologic stress agent.
- ☐ Assess for pregnancy and breastfeeding.
- ☐ Obtain a signed consent form.
- ☐ Add other patient preparations as appropriate

DOSAGE

1. Technetium-99m product name administered via intravenous injection:_____
2. Rest: [value] _____mCi
3. Stress: [value] _____ mCi
☐ 90-100 minutes must pass between Rest injection and stress injection
☐ *Two-Day Stress/Rest Tc99m 24 hours must pass between Rest injection and stress injection
☐ [Weight adjusting chart may be attached if applicable]

_____

4. Non-radioactive drugs—Aminophylline:
5. Dose: [value]_____ mg
6. Intravenous infusion
7. Timing of administration: [value]_____
8. Precautions/Restrictions: [value]_____

ADENOSINE STRESS PATIENTS ONLY:

6. Non-radioactive drugs—Aminophylline:
7. Dose: [value] __ mg
8. Intravenous infusion
9. Timing of administration:
    ____[value] If needed wait 2 minutes after Myoview injection to give Aminophylline
10. Precautions/Restrictions: [value] Do not give to patients allergic to Xanthines

CAMERA/COMPUTER SETUP
ACQUISITION & PROCESSING PROTOCOLS
CAMERA MAKE MODEL:

EMERGENCY SHUT DOWN OF EQUIPMENT:

Camera setup (collimator, energy window setting, etc)

Patient and camera positioning

Camera/computer specific acquisition protocols including timing of views, time/counts per view, number of views as well as specific parameters and filtering including orbit, number of stops, time per stop, ECG-gating set-up

Camera/computer specific processing and reconstruction protocols, including standards for filtering

Camera/computer specific display protocols

Appropriate image labeling instruction - including name, patient identification, date and type of study, time interval as appropriate, view or projection and anatomical markers as appropriate

	REST STUDY	STRESS STUDY
Minimum time interval between rest and stress studies		
Time interval between tracer injection and imaging		
Energy		
Matrix		
Pixel size		
Number of projections		
Orbit		
Start angle		
End angle		
Time per view		
Gating		
Gating bins		
R to R window		
Uniformity and COR		
Prefilters		
Filter cutoff/power		
Motion correction		
Attenuation correction		
Normal database		
Reconstruction filter		

[If the acquisition, processing, or display protocols are predefined within your computer software, ICANL allows these to be listed as such in this document, and a copy of the applicable protocol from the manufacturer's procedure manual may be attached. However, for any portion of the procedure that requires user selection (time/view, filter cutoffs,), you must indicate your selections. You may use "Print Screen" while operating the computer software to show your selections.]

ARCHIVING
Indicate image-archiving procedures as appropriate

_____

_____

_____

STRESS PROCEDURE

For physical exercise:

The patient will be attached to a 12-lead ECG, and have an IV in place. The patient will go through a series of graded levels of exercise lasting 3 minutes each.

Enter modified protocol here]

- ☐ Record blood pressure, heart rate, and ECG every _____ minutes.
- ☐ The radiotracer should be injected at target heart rate and peak exercise 1 to 2 minutes prior to the conclusion of exercise.
- ☐ Record radiotracer injection time.
- ☐ The end point will be determined either by the patient's inability to continue or at the direction of the attending cardiologist supervising the study.
- ☐ Continue post-stress monitor of blood pressure, heart rate, and ECG for _____ minutes.
- ☐ Add indications for termination of exercise

_____

_____

_____

_____

FOR PHARMACOLOGIC STRESS:

- ☐ Pharmacologic stress agent:_____ name_____
- ☐ Method of administration _____
- ☐ Dosing:_____ Other consideration:_____
- ☐ Record blood pressure, heart rate, and ECG every _____ minutes.
- ☐ The radiotracer should be injected according to the applicable pharmacologic stress protocol.
- ☐ The end point will be determined by the completion of the pharmacologic stress agent administration following injection of the radiotracer.
- ☐ Continue post-stress monitoring of blood pressure, heart rate, and ECG for _____minutes after completion of the pharmacologic stress agent.
- ☐ ADVERSE REACTIONS:
- ☐ Minor side effects (flushing, chest pain, dyspnea, dizziness, nausea, symptomatic hypotension) are common and occur in approximately 80% of patients. Chest pain is non-specific and not necessarily indicative of the presence of CAD.
- ☐ High degree AV block occurs in ~7% of cases. ST-segment depression ≥1mm occurs in 15% to 20% of cases; however, unlike chest pain, this is indicative of significant CAD.
- ☐ Treatment of adverse reactions:
- ☐ Give aminophylline when indicated for symptoms. If clinically possible, this should be delayed until at least 2 minutes after radiotracer injection.

NUCLEAR MEDICINE
B2.2   Gated Equilibrium Radionuclide
Ventriculography (MUGA)

PROCEDURE:
Common Indications

Parameters obtained from RVG include the following:
1. Global ventricular systolic function
2. Regional wall motion
3. Ventricular volumes (qualitative or quantitative)
4. Responses of above parameters to exercise or other interventions
5. Systolic and diastolic function indices
6. Stroke volume ratios

Common clinical settings in which RVG may be useful include:
1. Known or suspected coronary artery disease (C A D)
        1.1.1. CAD without myocardial infarction (MI)
        1.1.2. Remote MI c. Acute MI (however, these patients usually should not undergo exercise stress in the first 48 hours after acute MI)
    1.2.   To help distinguish systolic from diastolic causes of congestive heart failure (CHF) in patients with known or suspected CHF
    1.3.   Evaluation of cardiac function in patients undergoing chemotherapy
    1.4.   Assessment of ventricular function in patients with valvular heart disease

An RVG may be used in the conditions listed above for (a) determining long-term prognosis; (b) assessing short-term risk (e.g., preoperative evaluation); and (c) monitoring response to surgery or other therapeutic interventions.

PATIENT PREPARATION
REST
No special preparation is required for a resting RVG. A fasting state is generally preferred. It is not necessary to withhold any medications. The electrodes used for cardiac gating must be placed securely on the skin to ensure an optimal ECG signal.

EXERCISE
1. The patient should be fasting for at least 3–4 hours before the study and should be both hemodynamically and clinically stable.
2. Exercise stress, in the form of supine or upright ergometry, is generally preferred. Patients who are unable to exercise for noncardiac reasons may undergo pharmacologic stress with a positive inotropic agent. It is recommended that medications that may alter the heart rate response be withheld unless medically contraindicated or the efficacy of the medication is being tested by the exercise test.

3. Life support instrumentation and cardiac resuscitative drugs must be available in the immediate vicinity of the stress laboratory. A physician or other personnel trained in advanced cardiac life support (ACLS) must be immediately available during the stress and recovery phases. Continuous, preferably 12-lead ECG monitoring must also be performed throughout all phases of the stress study.

4. Intermittent blood pressure measurement and ECG tracings should be performed before, during, and in the recovery phases of the stress study. The patient should be clinically observed during and immediately after the stress test. Any abnormalities in symptomatology, hemodynamics, or the ECG should be monitored until resolved.

INFORMATION PERTINENT TO PERFORMING THE PROCEDURE

1. An adequate history and cardiovascular examination should be obtained before diagnostic evaluation.
2. Specific areas to be reviewed include the indication(s) for testing, medications, symptomatology, cardiac risk factors, and prior cardiac procedures (diagnostic or therapeutic).
3. The patient's cardiac rhythm should be noted, because marked heart rate variability may limit the ability to both perform and interpret the RVG.
4. Physical limitations may limit or preclude the performance of a study requiring physical exercise. A resting 12-lead ECG should be reviewed before an exercise study.

PRECAUTIONS

1. It is mandatory that Occupational Safety and Health Administration guidelines for safe handling of human blood products be followed at all times when techniques labeling autologous RBCs are used.
2. When an in vitro method is used for radiolabeling autologous RBCs, a fail-safe policy and procedure must be in place and implemented to assure that administration of labeled cells to the wrong patient is prevented.
3. Patients with potentially unstable cardiac rhythms (e.g., paroxysmal supraventricular or ventricular tachycardia) or implanted devices (e.g., implantable defibrillators) may require special precautions, because heart rate response to exercise may be unpredictable.

RADIOPHARMACEUTICALS

1. For the adult, the usual administered activity is 555–1110 MBq (15–30 mCi) autologous RBCs labeled with Tc-99m using the in vivo, modified in vivo, or in vitro techniques.
2. The usual administered activity in children is 7–15 MBq/kg (0.2–0.4 mCi/kg), with a minimum dose of 70–150 MBq (2–4 mCi).
3. The largest absorbed radiation dose to an organ is that to the heart (about 0.02 mSv/MBq). Tc-99m–labeled RBCs distribute within the blood-pool with an estimated volume of distribution of approximately 4%–7% of body weight.
4. The estimated biological half-life is approximately 24–30 hours. Approximately 25% of the administered dose is excreted in the urine in the first 24 hours.
5. A stannous pyrophosphate preparation is typically used in most red cell labeling techniques. The dosage of this preparation may need to be increased in patients receiving "fulldose" heparin and in patients in renal failure.
6. Labeling is least consistent with the in vivo method, intermediate with the modified in vivo method, and most consistent with the in vitro method. Tc-99m–radiolabeled human serum albumin (HSA) is an alternative to radiolabeled RBCs. However, images are usually of lower quality because of the escape of tracer from the intravascular space and breakdown of the albumin, resulting in decreased contrast.

Radiation Dosimetry for Adults			
Radiopharmaceutical	Administered activity MBq (mCi)	Organ Receiving the largest radiation dose mGy per MBq (rad per mCi)	Effective dose mSv per MBq (rem per mCi)
Tc-99m labeled red blood cells[1]	555 – 1110 i.v. (15 – 30)	0.023 Heart 0.085	(0.085) (0.031)
Tc-99m albumin[2]	370 – 740 i.v. (10 – 20)	0.020 Heart (0.074)	0.0079 (0.029)
Radiation Dosimetry for Children 5-year-old			
Radiopharmaceutical	Administered activity MBq (mCi)	Organ Receiving the largest radiation dose mGy per MBq (rad per mCi)	Effective dose mSv per MBq (rem per mCi)
Tc-99m labeled red blood cells[1]	7 – 15 i.v. (0.2 – 0.4)	0.062 Heart (0.23)	0.025 (0.093)
Tc-99m albumin[2]	5 – 10 i.v. (0.1 – 0.3)	0.054 Heart (0.23)	0.023 (0.085)

IMAGE ACQUISITION
REST STUDY
Instrumentation
1. Acquisition is performed by a gamma camera interfaced to a dedicated computer. Images may be acquired with either a low-energy all-purpose (LEAP) or high-resolution parallel-hole collimator.
2. An appropriate ECG gating device should interface with the acquisition computer. The simultaneity of the gating device's R-wave trigger and the patient's QRS complex should be verified before initiation of the study.
3. An appropriate RR interval beat acceptance window should be selected to account for heart rate variability and ectopy.
4. Systolic function determinations are less susceptible to heart rate variability than diastolic function measurements. "List" mode acquisition is useful for making a composite cardiac cycle from a heterogenous population of beats and for retrograde gating for diastolic parameters.

ACQUISITION PARAMETERS
1. A minimum of 16 frames per R-R interval are required for an accurate assessment of ventricular wall motion and assessment of ejection fraction.

2. A higher framing rate (32–64 frames per R-R) is preferred for detailed measurement of diastolic filling parameters and is required for absolute volume measurements.

3. Acceptable indices of diastolic function are achievable at 16 frames per cardiac cycle, if Fourier curve fitting is employed.

4. Images should be acquired so that the heart occupies ~50% of the usable field of view.

5. Typical acquisitions are for a total of 3–7 million counts. Supine imaging is performed in a minimum of 3 views to visualize all wall segments of the left ventricle. The left anterior oblique (LAO) acquisition is obtained at 45° or at an angle that allows the best separation of the right and left ventricles (best septal or best separation view).

6. An anterior acquisition is obtained in a straight (0°) anterior projection or at an angle ~45° less than the "best septal" view.

7. The lateral acquisition is obtained as a left cross-table lateral or at an angle that is approximately 45° greater than the best septal view.

8. The lateral view may also be acquired in the right-sidedown left lateral decubitus position.

9. This altered positioning may improve visualization of the true posterobasal segment. A 70° LAO acquisition may be used instead of a left cross-table lateral view.

10. Left posterior oblique (LPO) or right anterior oblique (RAO) acquisitions may be of additional benefit.

11. These angles often need to be altered in patients with congenital heart or lung anomalies or right-sided overload. A slant-hole collimator may be used for angulation in the caudal–cephalic plane to help separate the ventricles from the atria.

STRESS STUDY
Instrumentation
    A high sensitivity or LEAP collimator is preferred for the stress equilibrium study.

ACQUISITION PARAMETERS
1. Sixteen frames per R-R interval are sufficient for assessment of ventricular wall motion and LVEF. SPECT imaging with 8 or 16 frames is an acceptable substitute.

2. Images may be acquired on a bicycle ergometer in either a supine, semiupright, or upright position using the best septal view as previously described or other views as appropriate to visualize a specific region of interest (ROI).

3. The most accurate determination of the LVEF is usually obtained in the best septal view.

4. Images may be acquired at multiple levels of exercise.
5. A 2–3-minute acquisition may be attained at each new level of exercise once a stable heart rate is attained (usually beginning after 1 minute of exercise at the new level).
6. The last stage of exercise may be extended to increase image statistics, but workload should not be decreased.
7. A postexercise RVG is desirable to assess postexercise recovery; LVEF increases promptly in the great majority of patients.
8. Pharmacologic stress with inotropic agents, mental stress, and atrial or ventricular pacing are other, less common alternatives to exercise testing.

INTERVENTIONS

Mental stress studies or pharmacologic stress as well as pacing are potential interventions in patients who cannot exercise.

PROCESSING

1. The cine loop should be reviewed for adequacy of counting statistics, appropriate ECG gating, adequacy of radiopharmaceutical labeling, and positioning of the heart.
2. A subjective visual assessment of left ventricular systolic function should be performed before calculation of LVEF.
3. ROIs should be created, either manually by the operator or automatically by the computer, so that all activity from the left ventricle is encompassed by the ROI.
4. The ROI used for background correction should be free of activity from the spleen or descending aorta. Other ventricular systolic and diastolic parameters may be generated.
5. Discrepancies between the calculated LVEF and qualitative left ventricular systolic function should be resolved by reprocessing, when necessary. Ventricular volumes may be calculated using either count-based or geometric methods.
6. Calculation of the stroke volume ratio may be helpful in patients suspected of valvular disease. Spatial and temporal filtering may be used, if desired, to enhance visual appearance of the images. Parametric images (e.g., phase/amplitude images) may also aid in image interpretation.

INTERPRETATION CRITERIA

1. Cardiac morphology
   1.1. The morphology, orientation, and sizes of the cardiac chambers and great vessels should be evaluated subjectively and reported. The thickness of the pericardial silhouette and the ventricular wall may also be evaluated subjectively and reported. When measured, absolute ventricular volumes may also be included, although measurements of absolute ventricular volumes by planar images are problematic. SPECT measurements will be more reliable. Automated programs to calculate ejection fraction and volumes are preferable for gated SPECT.
2. Systolic ventricular function

2.1.   Global left ventricular function should be assessed qualitatively and compared with the calculated ejection fraction. Discrepancies should be resolved by reprocessing, when necessary.

3. Normal values for LVEF range between ~50% and 80% at rest and between 56% and 86% at stress.

4. All left ventricular segments should be assessed for regional function using cinematic display of each view. Abnormalities of contraction should be described using the conventional terms of mild, moderate, or severe hypokinesia, akinesia, and dyskinesia. Systematic reporting may be aided by standardized recording forms. Parametric images, such as phase and amplitude images, may be useful in evaluating

5. regional variations in the timing and magnitude of contraction, identifying valve planes, and identification of conduction abnormalities.

6. The pattern of left ventricular diastolic function may be evaluated qualitatively from the volume curve and reported with quantitative measurements.

7. One can adjust for differences that result from heart rate or systolic function by dividing filling rate by emptying rate. Right ventricular systolic function may be approximated by calculation of RVEF; however, more accurate determination may require a different technique, such as first-pass RNA.

8. Normal values for RVEF range between ~46% and 70%.

9. Stress images

9.1.   The stress or intervention study should be displayed side-by-side with the resting study in cinematic mode. Changes in chamber sizes, regional wall motion, and global ejection fraction of both ventricles should be addressed qualitatively and reported with quantitative measures of ejection fraction.

10. Comparison with previous studies

10.1.   Results should be compared with any previous studies by direct comparison of the cinematic displays of the two studies, whenever possible. Discrepancies should be resolved by reprocessing when necessary.

REPORTING
PROCEDURES AND MATERIALS

1. Reporting of the method of ECG gating (forward only, buffered beat averaging), beat acceptance/ rejection, and underlying cardiac rhythm is optional. Type and dose of radiolabeling (Tc-99m RBCs in vivo, modified in vivo, in vitro; Tc-99m HSA) and views obtained should be reported.

FINDINGS

1. Cardiac morphology
2. Comment on size of various cardiac chambers, ventricular wall thickness and pericardial silhouette.
3. Systolic function
    3.1.   Report global LVEF.
    3.2.   Report regional left ventricular wall m o t i o n .
    3.3.   Option: report global RVEF.

3.4.   Option: report diastolic filling indices.

3.5.   Option: report systolic emptying indices.

4. Stress images

4.1.   Report baseline, peak and recovery L V E F .

4.2.   Report any alteration in visually assessed regional wall motion, global left and right ventricular function, a n d v o l u m e s .

4.3.   Option: report stress ECG and hemodynamics.

4.4.   Option: report left ventricular end-diastolic and end-systolic volume.

4.5.   Report noncardiac vascular abnormalities (e.g., aortic dilatation).

QUALITY CONTROL
SOURCES OF ERROR

1. RBC labeling

1.1.   Certain medications and disease processes (e.g., chronic renal failure) will decrease labeling efficiency and reduce the target-to background ratio.

2. Patient positioning

2.1.   The ejection fraction may be inaccurately calculated by inadequate separation of the left ventricle from other cardiac structures, especially the left atrium (which has time–activity curve that is the opposite of that of the left ventricle).

3. Gating errors

3.1.   A poor ECG signal or one in which complexes other than the QRS complex are dominant may result in spurious gating and data that are not interpretable.

3.2.   Care should be taken to ensure that the QRS complex is the triggering signal (e.g., choosing an ECG lead in which the QRS is much larger than the wave).

3.3.   The best gating can be obtained from systems that compute the rate of change of voltage on the ECG to be sure that the QRS and not the T wave is the signal used.

4. Heart rate variability

Significant heart rate variability may compromise the determination of diastolic filling indices.

5. Image statistics

Inadequate counts/frame may compromise image interpretation as well as decrease the statistical reliability of quantitative measurements.

6. Processing errors

Inclusion of nonventricular activity or exclusion of ventricular activity from ventricular ROIs may cause underestimation or overestimation of the ejection fraction. Including the left atrium in the ROI my also alter the LVEF. Inclusion of structures such as the spleen or the descending aorta in the background ROI may alter the LVEF.

7. Issues Requiring Further Clarification

None

NOTES

NUCLEAR MEDICINE
SECTION B2.2 DIAGNOSTIC IMAGING PROCEDURE PROTOCOLS

B2.2 ACC AHA 3-Lead Placement Diagram

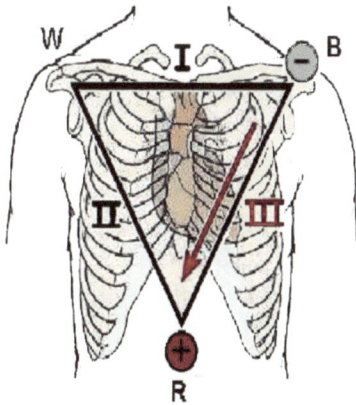

W – White Lead,
Always Negative Polarity

B- Black Lead,
Positive For Lead I,
Negative For Lead II

R – Red Lead,
Always Positive Polarity

Figure depicts the standard three-lead system that forms Einthoven's triangle. Note that while the red electrode is usually placed near the left lateral base of the chest; the electrical reference point for the red electrode tends to reside as shown. The arrow that is directed parallel to lead III represents a vector. If the wave of electrical depolarization moves parallel and in the same direction as this vector, the waveforms will be upright and the tallest in amplitude.

INSCRIPTION	COLOR	LOCATION
RA	WHITE	RIGHT ARM
LA	BLACK	LEFT ARM
RL	GREEN	RIGHT LEG
LL	RED	LEFT LEG
V1-6	BROWN	CHEST

- Try to keep the leads away from the area of the heart.
- Once the leads are connected to the patient, verify a valid ECG signal.
- If the R-wave signal is too low or R-wave detections is not consistent, move electrode RA toward the patient's left until the signal is acceptable.
- Make sure the lead cable will not move during the scan, possibly disconnection from the electrode.

NOTES:
The signal measured at RL is used as a measurement of the background
Due to variations in color-coding schemes for the lead cables, refer to the two letters engraved on the cables to identify the role of each lead.

NOTES

NUCLEAR MEDICINE
B2.2   Myoview Dobutamine Infusion Protocol

PURPOSE:
Alternative pharmacologic stress agent to increase myocardial perfusion without exercise and for patients that have drug intolerance, such as adenosine. Dobutamine can be used in patients exhibiting bronchospasm

PROCEDURE:
Absolute or relative Contraindications:
1. Severe arrhythmias
2. Psychiatric disorders

Patient Identification
1. Patient will check in at the front desk and the clerk will notify the Nuclear Medicine department.
2. The Nuclear Medicine Technologist will identify the patient by B2.1.1 Patient Identification Process
3. Two separate questions are to be asked.
    3.1.   State full name
    3.2.   State birth date

Patient Preparation:
1. Instructed to be NPO 4 hours prior to testing (a light caffeine-free breakfast is allowed depending on appointment time.
2. Beta-blockers (per ok with physician), and caffeine should be held for 24 hours prior to the dobutamine test.
3. The Nuclear Medicine technologist explains the test ot the patient and then obtains written consent.
4. An intravenous catheter is then inserted into a suitable antecubital vein using aseptic technique and universal precautions.
5. The Rest 10.0 mCi 99mTc-Myoview is the injected followed by three milliliters of normal saline.
6. Resting image are then acquired no sooner than 30 minutes later.

Dobutamine Stress Procedure:
1. Identify patient as above, full name and birth date.
2. A full explanation of the stress dobutamine test is given by the ACLS certified personnel performing the testing procedure, to include benefits, risks, and side effects.
3. A medical history form is completed to include a review of all medications.
4. The intravenous catheter is checked for patency.
5. The skin is prepped and electrodes are placed on the chest per ACC/AHA guidelines for stress testing(see attached diagram)
6. The patient is connected to the EKG/treadmill machine.

7. RN, physician, or ACLS certified individual will auscultate lung and heart sounds.
8. Resting EKG, HR, and Blood Pressure are recorded and used as a baseline.
9. Dobutamine is first diluted to a concentration of 1 mg/ml and in fused at incremental doses of 5, 10, 20, 30, and 40 ug/kg/min at 3 min intervals, until symptoms or attainment of target HR.
10. EKG tracings are recorded every 1-2 min and blood pressure is recorded every 3 minutes.
11. If target HR cannot be reached adjunctive small i.v. doses of Atropine, (0.25-0.50 mg/push should be used to reach the desired HR.
12. When the desired heart rate is achieved (MPHR) the 30.0mCi 99mTc-myoview can be injected followed by 3 milliliters of normal saline.
13. Patient should be monitored until HR, BP and respirations return to normal or baseline.
14. If blood pressure drops during infusion, simple leg elevation usually helps.
15. Occasionally, in the presence of sever symptoms-small doses of a beta blocker antidote may be need. This must first be approved by the cardiologist.
16. After full recovery of the patient and waiting at least 100 minutes between Rest injection and stress injection, the patient can now be scanned post stress.
17. Wait 30-60 minutes before scanning to allow biliary and intestinal activity to subside, this can be an adverse indication to proper imaging.
18. Imaging should be done according to the Gated Spect Imaging acquisition protocol and should not be edited in any way.

NUCLEAR MEDICINE
          B2.2   Dobutamine Stress Flow Sheet

PROCEDURE

NAME: _____

Add 250 mg of Dobutamine into 250 cc NS to get 1,000 mcg/cc solution.

Dosage calc: Pt.wt.(_____ kg/1000 mg/cc) x 60 gtt/min=_____ (l mcg/kg/min)

       (lmcg/kg/min) x 5mcg/kg/min= _____ (IVAC pump setting)
       x 10mcg/kg/min= _____
       x 20mcg/kg/min= _____
       x 30mcg/kg/min= _____
       x 40mcg/kg/min= _____

       Dobutamine Lot# _____ Exp. Date _____ CVT's signature

       Atropine given IV mg. Lot# _____ Exp. Date _____

       Lopressor given IV _____ mg Lot# _____ Exp. Date _____

Physician's Signature _____

NUCLEAR MEDICINE

B2.2   Dobutamine Dose Infusion Chart

Dobutamine 250mg in 250ccNS (mcg/kg/min)- value in cc/hr					
Weight(lbs)	5	10	20	30	40
100	13.6	27.3	54.5	81.8	109.1
105	14.3	28.6	57.3	85.9	114.5
110	15.0	30.0	60.0	90.0	120.0
115	15.7	31.4	62.7	94.1	125.5
120	16.4	32.7	65.5	98.2	130.9
125	17.0	34.1	68.2	102.3	136.4
130	17.7	35.5	70.9	106.4	141.8
135	18.4	36.8	73.6	110.5	147.3
140	19.1	38.2	76.4	114.5	152.7
145	19.8	39.5	79.1	118.6	158.2
150	20.5	40.9	81.8	122.7	163.6
155	21.1	42.3	84.5	126.8	169.1
160	21.8	43.6	87.3	130.9	174.5
165	22.5	45.0	90.0	135.0	180.0
170	23.2	46.4	92.7	139.1	185.5
175	23.9	47.7	95.5	143.2	190.9
180	24.5	49.1	98.2	147.3	196.4
185	25.2	50.5	100.9	151.4	201.8
190	25.9	51.8	103.6	155.5	207.3
195	26.6	53.2	106.4	159.5	212.7
200	27.3	54.5	109.1	163.6	218.2
205	28.0	55.9	111.8	167.7	223.6
210	28.6	57.3	114.5	171.8	229.1
215	29.3	58.6	117.3	175.9	234.5
220	30.0	60.0	120.0	180.0	240.0
225	30.7	61.4	122.7	184.1	245.5
230	31.4	62.7	125.5	188.2	250.9
235	32.0	64.1	128.2	192.3	256.4
240	32.7	65.5	130.9	196.4	261.8
245	33.4	66.8	133.6	200.5	267.3
250	34.1	68.2	136.4	204.5	272.7
255	34.8	69.5	139.1	208.6	278.2
260	35.5	70.9	141.8	212.7	283.6
265	36.1	72.3	144.5	216.8	289.1
270	36.8	73.6	147.3	220.9	294.5
275	37.5	75.0	150.0	225.0	300.0
280	38.2	76.4	152.7	229.1	305.5
285	38.9	77.7	155.5	233.2	310.9
290	39.5	79.1	158.2	237.3	316.4
295	40.2	80.5	160.9	241.4	321.8
300	40.9	81.8	163.6	245.5	327.3

NUCLEAR MEDICINE
      B2.2   Myoview Screening Questionnaire

Nuclear Medicine Department
Pregnancy Screening Questionnaire
(To be completed by female patients between the ages of 12 and 50)

       It is not known whether MYOVIEW, a diagnostic radiopharmaceutical imaging agent, can cause fetal harm when administered to a pregnancy woman, or can affect reproductive capacity. Medications typically do not present a significant risk to a developing fetus, or reduce the probability of carrying the fetus to term. There IS, however, no evidence that there is a "zero risk". Therefore, I understand it is important to determine if: "I am pregnant", "I do not think I am pregnant", or "I cannot be pregnant". Please assist us by checking the appropriate box below and sign below were indicated.

    ☐ I do not think I am pregnant (it has been 10 days or less since my last normal menstrual period.)

    ☐ I cannot be pregnant (i.e. no sexual activity, hysterectomy, bilateral tubal ligation, taking birth control pills and not missed any, menopause, or have not yet started having periods).

_____   _____
Witness Signature   Patient Signature

PATIENTS WHO ARE PREGNANT

After discussion with Dr. _____, and understanding the nature and purpose of the procedure, possible risks and precautions that will be taken:

    ☐ **I prefer to postpone the procedure.**

    ☐ **I want to undergo the procedure.**

_____   _____
Witness Signature   **Patient Signature**

NOTES

INSERT FACILITY PROTOCOL

B2.2   FACILITY DIAGNOSTIC IMAGING PROTOCOL

Page #

NUCLEAR MEDICINE
B2.3   Myocardial Perfusion Exercise Stress with Bruce Protocol

PURPOSE
To establish guidelines for the exercise portion of nuclear cardiology procedures.

PROCEDURE:
A treadmill exercise stress test is indicated to determine the presence of stress-induced myocardial ischemia; evaluate the potential for rhythm disturbance; determine the patient's blood pressure response to exercise; to evaluate the patient's exercise tolerance, and to provide an objective basis for an exercise prescription.

Absolute Contraindications:
1. Chest pain consistent with unstable angina.
2. Back or leg injuries or severe handicap that precludes use of the treadmill.
3. Decompensated or inadequately controlled CHF.
4. Uncontrolled blood pressure (e.g. resting BP >200/115 mmHg).
5. Acute myocardial infarction within last 2-3 days.
6. Severe pulmonary hypertension.
7. Uncontrolled cardiac arrhythmias.
8. Acute PE.
9. Unwillingness to give consent.
10. Acute myocarditis, endocarditis, pericarditis.

Relative Contraindications:
1. Severe aortic stenosis.
2. Hypertrophic obstructive cardiomyopathy.
3. Patients with LBBB or A-V paced rhythm.

Patient Identification:
1. Patient will check in at the front desk and the clerk will notify the Nuclear Medicine Department.
2. The Nuclear Technologist will identify patient according to the *B2.1.1   Patient Identification Process*
3. The Nuclear Technologist will assess all females for pregnancy and/or breastfeeding protocol (see Section2.1.2 Pregnancy/Breastfeeding Screening Protocol.
4. The Nuclear Technologist will confirm patient identity and verify appropriateness of exam according to the written order.

Patient Preparation:

☐ Patients are instructed to be NPO 4 hours prior to testing (a light caffeine-free breakfast is allowed depending on appointment time).

☐ Beta Blockers (per physician request) and caffeine are held for 24 hours prior to the test.

☐ The Nuclear Technologist explains the test to the patient and obtains written consent.

☐ A hep-lock is established preferably in an antecubital vein using aseptic technique and a rest Cardiolite 10.0 mCi dose is injected IV. Resting images are obtained no sooner than 30 minutes later (see Rest MPI protocol 2.2 Diagnostic Imaging Procedure Protocols).

☐ One Day Protocol: Inject the rest isotope dose followed by a 10cc saline flush.

☐ Resting images are obtained 30-45 minutes later. No sooner than 90 minutes post rest isotope injection, the patient is brought into the treadmill room.

☐ Two-Day Protocol: Stress test is performed first.

☐ A full explanation of the stress procedure is given by the RN or NP, including benefits, risks, and side effects.

☐ A medical history form is completed to include review of all medications.

☐ The heparin well is checked for patency. Skin is prepped and electrodes are placed on the chest per ACC/AHA guidelines for stress testing (see attached diagram).

☐ The patient is connected to the EKG/treadmill machine. Resting EKG's are obtained and used as the baseline.

☐ Resting blood pressure is also taken.

☐ The supervising NP, RN, or physician will auscultate lung and heart sounds.

☐ Demonstrate on how to walk on the treadmill.

☐ Under NP, RN, or physician supervision, *Bruce protocol is performed where the speed and incline are increased every three minutes as follows:

Stage	Speed (mph)	Grade	Time	METs
Rest	1.2	0.00	0	1.9
1	1.7	10.0	3:00	4.6
2	2.5	12	6:00	7.0
3	3.4	14	9:00	10.1
4	4.2	16	12:00	12.9
5	5	18	15:00	15.0
6	5.5	20	18:00	16.9

1. Exercise is continued until the patient's maximum effort is achieved, or until one of the following Endpoints indicates early termination of exercise:
    1.1. Maximum heart rate is achieved.
    1.2. Marked ischemic changes are present (>3mm St segment depression).
    1.3. Ischemic ST segment elevation (>1mm in leads without pathological Q waves).
    1.4. Severe chest pain, marked dyspnea or dizziness.
    1.5. Systolic blood pressure exceeds 230 mmHg or 130 mmHg diastolic.
    1.6. Decrease in Systolic BP >20 mmHg from the resting BP.
    1.7. Presence of ventricular tachycardia (VT), or supraventricular tachycardia (SVT).
    1.8. NP, RN, or physician terminates the test at his/her discretion.

2. Injection Criteria: At peak stress, as determined per the NP, RN, or physician, the stress dose of Cardiolite 30.0 mCi is administered through the heparin well. Goal is 85% MPHR (MPHR, defined as 220-age). If no EKG changes are noted and no chest pain, the patient should exercise to patient's maximum capacity. Inject patient with 30.0 mCi two minutes before stopping treadmill.
3. Patient is instructed to continue exercising for 2 minutes post isotope injection. Note: If that target heart rate is not achieved, the test may be changed to a pharmacological stress at the supervising physician's discretion.
4. Monitoring is continuous throughout the test by the supervising physician. EKG's and blood pressures are taken at a minimum of once each exercise state.

Post-stress monitoring
1. Once exercise is terminated the patient sits down, additional twelve lead EKG's and blood pressures are recorded every one to two minutes for a minimum of 6 minutes. Any ischemic changes or symptoms must be resolved, and the heart rate and blood pressure must return to baseline before the patient is disconnected.
2. If the patient is deemed stable pr the supervising NP, RN, or physician, the heparin well is removed and placed in hot trash.
3. The patient is shown the waiting room or holding area to await post-stress imaging.
4.

Treatment of Adverse Effects (at physician's discretion)

1. Per NP, or physician order, unresolved chest pain may be treated with sublingual Nitroglycerin or IV Metoprolol.
2. Unresolved symptomatic hypotension
    2.1. Place patient in Trendelenburg position and/or bolus IV fluids per physician order.
    2.2. If severe hypotension is still present patient should be sent to the ER.
3. Onset of sustained arrhythmia
    3.1. Have patient cough or perform Valsalva maneuver.
    3.2. If patient remains unstable, treat by activating ACLS procedures.
    3.3. Transport to ER.

SPECIAL INSTRUCTIONS:

1. Any caffeine is held 24 hours prior to the test, including decaffeinated beverages (coffee, tea, sodas, chocolates, and some aspirin).
2. Comfortable clothing should be worn to walk on a treadmill (sneakers, light clothing).
3. Beta Blockers ideally are held for 24 hours prior to testing, unless otherwise directed by the physician.
4. Patients should not eat or drink anything 4 hours prior to the test.
5. Insulin dependent diabetic patients may take ½ of their insulin dose with a light snack 2 hours prior to testing.

NUCLEAR MEDICINE
    B2.3   Bruce/Modified/Low Chart

BRUCE PROTOCOL

STAGE	SPEED (Mph)	GRADE (%)	DURATION (min: sec)	METS
Rest				
1	1.7	10.0	3:00	4.6
2	2..5	12 .0	3:00	7.0
3	3.4	14.0	3:00	10.1
4	4.2	16	3:00	12.9
5	5.0	18.0	3:00	15.0
6	5.5	20.0	3:00	16.9
7	6.0	22.0	3:00	19.1
Recovery	0.0	0.0	6:00	…

MODIFIED BRUCE PROTOCOL

STAGE	SPEED (Mph)	GRADE (%)	DURATION (min: sec)	METS
Rest	0.0	0.0	…	…
1	1.2	0.0	3:00	1.9
2	1.7	0.0	3:00	2.3
3	1.7	5.0	3:00	3.5
4	1.7	12.0	3:00	4.6
5	2.5	14.0	3:00	7.0
6	3.4	16.0	3:00	12.9
7	4.2	18.0	3:00	15.0
8	5.0	20.0	3:00	16.9
9	5.5	22.0	3:00	19.1
Recovery	0.0	0.0	6:00	…

LOW LEVEL PROTOCOL

STAGE	SPEED (Mph)	GRADE (%)	DURATION (min: sec)	METS
Rest	0.0	0.0	…	…
1	1.2	0.0	3:00	1.9
2	1.2	3.0	3:00	2.4
3	1.7	6.0	3:00	3.7
4	1.7	6.0	3:00	3.7
5	1.7	10.0	3:00	4.6
6	2.5	12.0	3:00	7.0
Recovery	0.0	0.0	6:00	…

NOTES

NUCLEAR MEDICINE
SECTION B2.3 STRESS PROCEDURES PROTOCOLS

B2.3 12-   ACC AHA Lead Placement Diagram

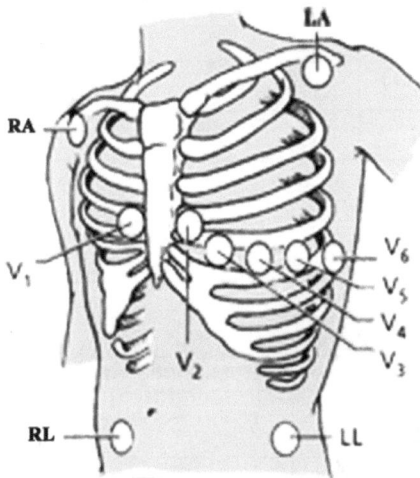

∴ **Note: Arm leads may be moved laterally to avoid excess motion artifact.**

1. Right and Left arm leads should be placed outwardly on the shoulder, preferentially over bone rather than muscle
2. V1 and V2 are positioned in the fourth intercostals space
3. Right leg lead (ground lead) should be placed below the umbilicus
4. V4 should be placed in the 5th intercostals space on the mid-clavicular line
5. V3 lies halfway between V2 and V4
6. V4, V5, V6, should be placed along a horizontal line, this line does not necessarily follow the intercostals space (V6 Mid-axillary)
7. The left leg lead should be just below the umbilicus

NUCLEAR MEDICINE

B2.3   Adenosine Cardiolite Stress Chart

PATIENT		DATE			
AGE		REFERRED BY			
SEX		INTERPRETED BY			
WEIGHT	*POUNDS*	PROTOCOL			
INDICATION		HEART RATE		TARGET	MAX
REST	mCi CARDIOLITE				
STRESS	mCi CARDIOLITE	CARDIAC MEDS			

MINUTES	HR	BP	SYMPTOMS	ARRHYTHMIAS	FLAT/DOWN SLOPING ST DEPRESSION (mm)
Baseline					
1.					
2.					
3.					
4.					
5.					
6.					
7.					
8.					
9.					
10.					
11.					
12.					
13.					
14.					
15.					

Aminophylline Administered   ☐Yes _____ ☐No _____

Aminophylline Administered   _____mg

Accepted by: _____ (Initials) Date_____   .

NUCLEAR MEDICINE

B2.3   Cardiolite Treadmill EKG Chart

PATIENT		DATE		
AGE		REFERRED BY		
SEX		INTERPRETED BY		
WEIGHT	*POUNDS*	PROTOCOL		
INDICATION		HEART RATE	TARGET	MAX
REST	mCi CARDIOLITE			
STRESS	mCi CARDIOLITE	CARDIAC MEDS		

EXERCISE

MINUTES REST	HR	BP	SYMPTOMS	ARRHYTHMIAS	COMMENTS
16.					
17.					
18.					
19.					
20.					
21.					
22.					
23.					
24.					
25.					
26.					
27.					

RECOVERY

MINUTE REST	HR	BP	SYMPTOMS	ARRHYTHMIAS	COMMENT
1.					
2.					
3.					
4.					
5.					
6.					
7.					
8.					
9.					
10.					
11.					
12.					

OBSERVATIONS   Injections Time _____

Exercise Time_____

Max Heart Rate_____

METS_____% of heart rate achieved _____

CONCLUSIONS:_____

NUCLEAR MEDICINE
B2.3   Six Minute Adenosine Stress Protocol

PURPOSE:
To visualize perfusion and function of the myocardium when evaluating a patient for coronary artery disease who is physically not able to perform on a treadmill.

PROCEDURE:
An Adenosine stress test is used to determine the presence of myocardial ischemia or infarction in those patients who are unable to exercise adequately, have a paced rhythm or a LBBB, have a blunted heart rate response due to beta block, or are S/P acute MI (<3 days) and angioplasty/stenting (<2 weeks). The mechanism of action for adenosine is increasing the extravascular concentration of adenosine.

Absolute Contraindications:
1. Reactive airway disease (COPD emphysema, asthma) with active bronchospasm/wheezing. *See below
2. Use of Dipyridamole or Xanthine derivatives in the last 24 hours.
3. Recent hospitalization or intubation due to lung disease.
4. Sick sinus syndrome, and Second or third degree AV block without a pacemaker.
5. Hypotension (resting systolic <90 mm Hg.)
6. Acute MI (less than 48 hours)
7. Unstable angina
8. Unwillingness to give consent

Relative Contraindications:
1. Controlled asthma or current medical treatment inhalers (at physician's discretion)*
2. History of mild COPD or Emphysema*
3. Severe sinus bradycardia (heart rate<40 bpm)

Patient Identification:
1. Patient will check in at the front desk and the clerk will notify the Nuclear Medicine Department.
2. The Nuclear Technologist will identify patient according to B2.1.1 Patient Identification Process
3. The Nuclear Technologist will assess all females for pregnancy and/or breastfeeding protocol (see Section 2.1.2 Pregnancy/Breastfeeding Screening Protocol.
4. The Nuclear Technologist will confirm patient identity and verify appropriateness of exam according to the written order.
5. Ask Patient to:
   - 5.1.   State Full Name
   - 5.2.   State Birth Date

Patient Preparation:

1. Patients are instructed to be NPO 4 hrs. Prior to testing (a light caffeine-free breakfast is allowed depending on appointment time).
2. The Nuclear Technologist explains the test to the patient and obtains written consent.
3. A HEP-lock is established preferably in an antecubital vein using aseptic technique and a rest Myoview dose is injected IV. Resting images are obtained no sooner than 30 minutes later (see Rest MPI protocol).
4. One Day Protocol: Inject the rest isotope dose followed by a 10 cc saline flush.
5. Resting images are obtained 30-45 minutes later. No sooner than 90 minutes post rest isotope injection, the patient is brought into the treadmill room.
6. A full explanation of the stress procedure is given by the RN or NP, including benefits, risks, and side effects.
7. A medical history form is completed to include review of all medications.
8. The heparin well is check for patency. Skin is prepped and electrodes are placed on the chest per ACC/AHA guidelines for stress testing (see attached diagram).
9. The patient is connected to the EKG/treadmill machine. Resting EKG's are obtained and used as the baseline.
10. Resting Blood pressure is also taken.
11. The supervising NP, RN, or physician will auscultate lung and heart sounds.
12. Adenoscan is prepared by the local radiopharmacy according to the patient's weight in kg and calculating the dose by using the formula below, or by following the 6-minute chart.
13. Adenosine Dose Calculation:
14. Pt wt (lbs) _____ divided by 2.2 = _____ kg X 0.140
15. mg/kg/min = _____ mg/min _____ mg/min X 6 min = _____ total
16. mg divided by 3 = _____ total ml Adenosine
17. BAXA pump/60cc syringe: The weight-based Adenoscan dose is calculated and drawn into the 60cc syringe and labeled with name, date, and dose.
18. After package check in per protocol, the unit dose is verified for pharmaceutical type, expiration date, patient name, and amount of dose.
19. Connect a microbore extension tubing to the end of the syringe and connect a Y-connector to the end of the tubing and prime.
20. Under NP, RN, or physician supervision, press "Start" on the pump at the same time as the test/treadmill is started on the EKG/treadmill machine. Adenosine is administered at a rate of 140/ug/kg/min (Rabbit Setting) for six minutes in conjunction with low-level exercise (1-1.7 mph, 0% grade). If patient is unable to walk steadily, arm exercise or leg lifts may be used. In the presence of ventricular pacing, or LBBB, exercise is not performed.
21. Injection Criteria: Three minutes after the start of the adenosine infusion a stress Myoview dose is administered IV via the 2nd port of the Y-connector. The adenosine continues to infuse for 2 more minutes.

22. Monitoring: EKG's and blood pressures are taken every one to two minutes during infusion and into the recovery phase.

23. Post-stress monitoring: In the recovery phase, the patient is monitored for a minimum of 2 minutes and until symptoms, blood pressure, and/or ischemic EKG changes are resolved per NP, RN, or physician's discretion.

24. Early Endpoints: Per Adenoscan manufacturer recommendations, the first course of action in patients that are very symptomatic should be to titrate the dose down to a rate of 100ug/kg/min (Turtle Setting) with the injection occurring at the midway point based on total volume. Early termination of the Adenosine infusion may occur during the following instances: Severe hypotension (<80mm Hg), symptomatic persistent 2nd or 3rd degree heart block, wheezing, or severe chest pain with <2 mm ST depression.

25. If the patient is deemed stable per the supervising NP, RN, or physician, the IV and Y-connector are removed and placed in hot trash.

26. Gated stress images are obtained at a minimum of 30 minutes. 100 minutes must past between rest injection and stress injection.

Emergency Management

1. Crash cart must be nearby.
2. Treat arrhythmias per Physician order and ACLS protocol.
3. Patients with unresolved symptomatic hypotension, should be placed in Trendelenburg position and/or have IV fluids administered per physician order.
4. Due to the short half-life of Adenoscan (<10 sec.), most severe side effects resolve on their own. However, if early termination of the infusion occurs, and the patient experiences severe dyspnea, bronchospasm, or significant wheezing, it may be necessary to give up to 125 mg. Aminophylline SLOW (IV) over 2 minutes per physician order. May repeat additional 125 mg. doses per physician order. Note: Observe for Aminophylline-induced arrhythmias. Physician should be present until Aminophylline is administered and available for 15 minutes thereafter.
5. Persistent breathing difficulties post-Adenoscan infusion can also be treated with an Albuterol inhaler per physician order.

Special Instructions:

1. Comfortable clothing should be worn to walk on a treadmill (sneakers, light clothing).
2. Patients should not eat or drink anything 4 hours prior to the test.
3. Any caffeine is held 24 hours prior to the test, including decaffeinated beverages (coffee, tea, sodas, chocolates, and some aspirin).
4. Insulin dependent diabetic patients may take ½ of their insulin dose with a light snack 2 hours prior to testing.
5. Xanthene derivatives should be held 48 hours prior to test day.
6. Aggrenox to be held 2-3 days prior to test day.

NUCLEAR MEDICINE

B2.3   Adenoscan Appropriate Infusion p/Body Weight   30 mg. = 1 unit

PATIENT WEIGHT		INFUSION RATE	Total Volume Over 6 Min		
kg	lbs	ml/min	mL	TOTAL MG	UNITS
45	99	2.1	12.6	37.8	
46	101	2.1	12.9	38.7	
47	103	2.2	13.2	39.6	
48	106	2.2	13.4	40.2	
49	108	2.3	13.7	41.1	
50	110	2.3	14.0	42.0	
51	112	2.4	14.3	42.9	
52	114	2.4	14.6	43.8	
53	117	2.5	14.8	44.4	2 UNITS
54	119	2.5	15.1	45.3	
55	121	2.6	15.4	46.2	
56	123	2.6	15.7	47.1	
57	125	2.7	16.0	48.0	
58	128	2.7	16.2	48.6	
59	130	2.8	16.5	49.5	
60	132	2.8	16.8	50.4	
61	134	2.8	17.1	51.3	
62	136	2.9	17.4	52.2	
63	139	2.9	17.6	52.8	
64	141	3.0	17.9	53.7	
65	143	3.0	18.2	54.6	
66	145	3.1	18.5	55.5	
67	147	3.1	18.8	56.4	
68	150	3.2	19.0	57.0	
69	152	3.2	19.3	57.9	
70	154	3.3	19.6	58.8	
71	156	3.3	19.9	59.7	
72	158	3.4	20.2	60.6	3 UNITS
73	161	3.4	20.4	61.2	
74	163	3.5	20.7	62.1	
75	165	3.5	21.0	63.0	
76	167	3.5	21.3	63.9	
77	169	3.6	21.6	64.8	
78	172	3.6	21.8	65.4	
79	174	3.7	22.1	66.3	
80	176	3.7	22.4	67.2	

PATIENT WEIGHT		INFUSION RATE	Total Volume Over 6 Min		
81	178	3.8	22.7	68.1	
82	180	3.8	23.0	69.0	
83	183	3.9	23.2	69.6	
84	185	3.9	23.5	70.5	
85	187	4.0	23.8	71.4	
86	189	4.0	24.1	72.3	
87	191	4.1	24.4	7~"~	
88	194	4.1	24.6	73.8	
89	196	4.2	24.9	74.7	
90	198	4.2	25.2	75.6	
91	200	4.2	25.5	76.5	
92	202	4.3	25.8	77.4	
93	205	4.3	26.0	78.0	
94	207	4.4	26.3	78.9	
95	209	4.4	26.6	79.8	
96	211	4.5	26.9	80.7	
97	213	4.5	27.2	81.6	
98	216	4.6	27.4	82.2	
99	218	4.6	27.7	83.1	
100	220	4.7	28.0	84.0	
101	222	4.7	28.3	84.9	
102	224	4.8	28.6	85.8	
103	227	4.8	28.8	86.4	
104	229	4.9	29.1	87.3	
105	231	4.9	29.4	88.2	
106	233	4.9	29.7	89.1	
107	235	5.0	30.0	90.0	
108	238	5.0	30.2	90.6	4
109	240	5.1	30.5	91.5	U N I T S
110	242	5.1	30.8	92.4	

NUCLEAR MEDICINE
SECTION B2.3 STRESS PROCEDURES PROTOCOLS
List of Caffeine Products

POLICY:

The following products contain caffeine and should be withdrawn for 24 hours prior to stress testing:

- ☐ Coffee – both caffeinated or decaffeinated
- ☐ Tea – both caffeinated or decaffeinated
- ☐ Cocoa
- ☐ Chocolate Milk
- ☐ Milk chocolate, dark chocolate, and semi-sweet chocolate
- ☐ Baking chocolate
- ☐ Chocolate syrup
- ☐ Any dessert, ice cream, or any other food containing chocolate
- ☐ Any soft drinks – both caffeinated or decaffeinated
- ☐ Over the counter drugs – Anacin, Excedrin, or No-Doze
- ☐ Prescribed drugs – Cafergot, Darvon compounds, Fiorinal, Synalgos-DCM Wigraine
- ☐ _____
- ☐ _____
- ☐ _____
- ☐ _____

NUCLEAR MEDICINE
SECTION B2.3 STRESS PROCEDURES PROTOCOLS
Medications that Interfere

PROCEDURE:

The following products may need to be held prior to stress testing.   Please contact the office if you are currently taking any of these drugs:

HOLD PRIOR TO STRESS TESTING	
☐ Inderal	☐ Theovent Long Acting
☐ Lopressor	☐ Slo-bid Gyrocaps
☐ Tenormin	☐ Theospan-SR
☐ Toprol XL	☐ Theobid Jr Duracap
☐ Propanolol	☐ Theophylline SR
☐ Metoprolol	☐ Slo-Phylline Gyrocaps
☐ Atenolol	☐ Quibrin-T/SR
☐ Bisoprolo	☐ Theolair-SR
☐ Timolol	☐ Respid
☐ Cartelol	☐ Theo-24, Theo-Dur
☐ Betaxolol	☐ Persantine (Dipyridamole)
☐ Penbutolol	☐ Theoclear LA
☐ Zebeta	☐ Bronkodyl
☐ Ziac	☐ Sustaire
☐ Blocadren	☐ Uniphyl
☐ Cartrol	☐ Theo-Dur Sprinkle
☐ Kerlone	☐ Elixophyllin SR
☐ Levatol	☐ Constant-T
☐ Darvocet	☐ Aerolate
☐ Aggrenox	☐ Theochron
☐	☐
☐	☐
☐	☐
☐	☐
☐	☐
☐	☐

NUCLEAR MEDICINE

B2.4.2 PATIENT EDUCATION INSTRUCTIONS

Patients have been instructed about any food or diet restrictions. *Add department procedure (NPO or light meal) including number of hours prior to exam*

_____

_____

Patients should avoid foods containing caffeine for 24 hours prior to the stress study. These include:

- ☐ Chocolate and cocoa
- ☐ Coffee and tea to include any decaffeinated brands
- ☐ Colas or any drinks containing caffeine, including those with "caffeine-free" labels
- ☐ Aspirin containing caffeine
- ☐ Indicate other food or diet restrictions as appropriate

_____

_____

In consultation with the referring physician, consider discontinuation of specific medications prior to the procedure. Depending on the indication for stress testing and the clinical question to be answered, it may be advisable to discontinue certain medications. Patients should be instructed about withholding medications.

_____

_____

Include patient instruction sheet

PATIENT PREPARATION – FIRST DAY OF TEST
- ☐ Procedure and possible side effects of pharmacologic stress agent explained.
- ☐ Assess for pregnancy and breastfeeding.
- ☐ Signed consent form.
- ☐ Add other patient preparations as appropriate

_____

_____

DOSAGE
- ☐ Technetium-99m ____product name administered via intravenous injection:
- ☐ Stress: _____ mCi
- ☐ Rest: _____ mCi
- ☐ Weight adjusting chart may be attached if applicable
- ☐ Non-radioactive drugs—Aminophylline:
- ☐ Dose: _____ mg
- ☐ Intravenous infusion
- ☐ Timing of administration:_____
- ☐ Precautions/Restrictions: _____

NOTES

INSERT FACILITY SPECIFIC PROTOCOLS

MANUFACTURER SPECIFIC INSTRUCTIONS

Page #

NUCLEAR MEDICINE
B3.2   Imaging Equipment Quality Control Guideline

TEST (SCINTILLATION CAMERAS)		
PROCEDURE	**FREQUENCY**	**REFERENCE STANDARDS**
Collimator uniformity	Annually	Visually inspect for collimator defects
Energy Peaking	Daily (Prior To Use; Documentation Not Required)	Automatically done internally
Uniformity check A. Extrinsic (2-5 million counts)	A. Daily (prior to use)	3% = excellent 3-4% = good 4-5% = acceptable Above 6% = calibrate detector
COR Check	Weekly	X errors: Mean = -2 to +2 Max <4.6mm Min >-4.6mm Range <4.6mm / Y errors: Max <4.6mm Min >-4.6mm Range <4.6mm
QC Resolution Extrinsic (Bar Phantom)	Weekly	Visually Inspect all lines for full resolution
CALIBRATION		
High count calibration floods (>30 million count)	Monthly, Or Per Manufacturer's Recommendations	Compensates for non-uniformity
Center of rotation calibration (COR)	Monthly	Corrects for minor misalignment.
PM Tube Tuning	As necessary determined by uniformity check & monthly	Corrects gain for individual PM tubes that have drifted
PREVENTATIVE MAINTENANCE	Every 6 Months, Or Per Manufacturer's Recommendations	
PM tube check and tuning by service personnel	Quarterly	Manually inspect PM tubes and recalibrate them as needed to meet system guidelines
Collimator integrity	Annually	
Uniformity calibration	Per Manufacturer's Recommendations	

PROCEDURE:
COR (CENTER OF ROTATION)

STEP	DETAIL
1.	
2.	
3.	
4.	
5.	
6.	
7.	
8.	
9.	

RESOLUTION (BAR PHANTOM)

STEP	DETAIL
1.	
2.	
3.	
4.	
5.	
6.	
7.	
8.	
9.	
10.	

HIGH COUNT EXTRINSIC FLOOD

STEPS	DETAIL

UNIFORMITY CORRECTION

The uniformity of the scintillation crystal in the detector is dependant on the energy of the isotope used, and the collimators may have minor variations in sensitivit

INTRINSIC UNIFORMITY CALIBRATION

STEPS	DETAIL
1.	
2.	
3.	
4.	
5.	
6.	
7.	
8.	
9.	
10.	

EXTRINSIC UNIFORMITY CALIBRATION

STEPS	DETAIL
1.	
2.	
3.	
4.	
5.	
6.	
7.	
8.	
9.	
10.	
11.	
12.	
13.	
14.	
15.	

NUCLEAR MEDICINE

B3.2   Imaging Equipment Quality Control Log

DATE	FLOODS	BARS	COR	30M COUNT FLOOD	INITIALS

Accepted by: _____ (Initials) Date_____   .

NOTES

NUCLEAR MEDICINE
SECTION B3.3   NON-IMAGING QUALITY CONTROL

POLICY:
To establish guidelines for non-imaging quality control.
PROCEDURES:

DAILY DOSE CALIBRATOR_____:
1. Select "Test", daily
2. Background, enter, record value
3. Press Cs button
4. Check reading with 137 Cs source on 137Cs, 201Tl, and 99mTc settings.
5. Record all values in the Syntrac system *(If applicable)* or appropriate Quality Control form.

DAILY AREA SURVEYS _____:
1. Turn on GM meter.
2. Check battery.
3. Using pancake probe, record the source on the side of the meter.
4. Record a background reading.
5. Survey the following areas:
6. Camera Room 1 (to include table and keyboard)
7. Camera Room 2 (to include table and keyboard)
8. Injection Room.
9. Treadmill Room 1 (to include table, TM)
10. Hot Lab (to include dose prep, delivery area, and floor)
11. Cold trash
12. Waiting Area
13. Record all values in the Syntrac system *(If applicable)* or appropriate Quality Control form.

WEEKLY WIPE TESTS (LUDLUM 14C):
1. With an absorbent cotton swab, wipe the following areas and monitor at the surface of each wipe using the SM for contamination:
2. Dose Calibrator
3. Dose Calibrator Floor
4. Injection Chair
5. Injection Chair Floor
6. Camera
7. Camera Floor
8. Treadmill
9. Treadmill Floor
10. Hallway
11. Bathroom
12. Record all values in the Syntrac system *(If applicable)* or appropriate Quality Control form.

OTHER _____ :

1. _____
2. _____
3. _____
4. _____
5. _____
6. _____
7. _____
8. _____
9. _____
10. _____

QUARTERLY DOSE CALIBRATOR LINEARITY – CALI-CHECK TUBES METHOD:
This quality control test is completed by the contracted Health Physicist using the Cali-Check tubes.

1. Order a 99m Tc pre-calibrated source measuring at least 30mCi and place in DC.
2. Assay of activity at intervals of the source is measured inside each of the 12 tubes.
3. Results are calculated by the Health Physicist.
4. Results are entered into the Syntrac system *(If applicable)* record keeping.

Annual Dose Calibrator Accuracy:

5. This quality control test of the dose calibrator must be performed annually.
6. The Health Physicist performs this test at facility.
7. Use two sealed sources determined by the manufacturer to be within 5% of their state activity.
8. Decay each radionuclide to the present date and calculate upper and lower limits for the activity recorded.
9. Measure each sealed source twice and record values obtained.
10. Enter the values into the Syntrac system *(If applicable)* for linear accuracy or on the appropriate form.

ANNUAL SURVEY METER CALIBRATION:

1. The survey meter must be calibrated annually and is performed by the contracted Health Physicist.
2. Obtain a "loaner" survey meter from the contracted Health Physicist.
3. The survey meter in need of calibration is then sent to Health Physicist for calibration.
4. When calibration is complete, and the survey meter is returned, the "loaner" is then returned to the contracted Health Physicist.

NUCLEAR MEDICINE

B3.3.1   Inspection Equipment Testing Policy

POLICY:

To establish a procedure for the frequency requirements of Non-Imaging Quality Control

PROCEDURE:

Dose Calibrator Constancy	Daily
Area Survey including trash	Daily
Area Wipes	Weekly
Film Badge Record Review	Monthly
Sealed Source Inventory	Quarterly
Dose Calibrator Linearity	Quarterly
Radiation Safety Officer Review of Dose Calibrator, Linearity	Quarterly
Sealed Source Inventory, Area Surveys	Semi-Annually
Sealed Source Leak Test	Semi-Annually
Decontamination Kit Check	Semi-Annually
Radiation Safety In-service for Personnel	Annually
Procedure Manual Review	Annually
Survey Meter Calibration	Annually
Dose Calibrator Accuracy	Annually
Continuing Education	As Needed
Dose Calibrator Geometry	As Needed
License Renewal	As Needed
Postings	Duration of Authorized Use

Accepted by: _____ (Initials) Date_____   .

NOTES

NUCLEAR MEDICINE
B3.3.1   Hot Lab Equipment Calibration Protocol

POLICY:
To establish a procedure for calibration of hot lab equipment.

PROCEDURE:
Procedure for Calibrating Instruments Reading in mR/hr
Radiation survey meters will be calibrated with a radioactive source and an electronic pulser. When an electronic calibration is performed, the instrument will be checked for response to a radioactive source. Survey meters must be calibrated at least annually and after servicing (Battery changes are not considered "servicing".)

Survey meters will be function-tested with a check source or other dedicated source before each use. If the survey meter is not responding properly, radioactive material use must be suspended. There is no need to keep a record of these daily function checks.

1. The source must be approximately a point source when calibrating instruments reading in mR/hr.
2. The exposure rate at a given distance will be traceable by documented measurements to a standard certified within 5 percent accuracy by the National Institute of Standards and Technology (NIST).
3. The source will be of sufficient strength to give an exposure rate of approximately 30 mR/hr at 100 cm. Minimum activities of typical sources are 85 millicuries of Cs-137 or 21 millicuries of Co-60.
4. The inverse square law, transmission factors, and the radioactive decay law will be used to correct for change in exposure rate due to changes in distance, attenuation, or source decay.
5. A record will be made of each survey meter calibration.
6. A single point on a survey meter scale may be considered satisfactorily calibrated if the indicated exposure rate differs from the calculated exposure rate by less than 10 percent. If readings are between 10% and 20%, correction factors must be provided.
7. Readings above 1,000 mR/hr need not be calibrated.
8. At the time of calibration, the apparent exposure rate from a built-in or owner-supplied check source will be determined and recorded.
9. The report of the survey meter calibration will indicate the data obtained. This will include:
10. The owner or user of the instrument;
11. A description of the instrument that includes manufacturer, model number, serial number, and type of detector;
12. For each calibration point, the expected exposure rate, the measured exposure rate, and the scale selected on the instrument;

13. The angle between the radiation flux field and the detector (for external cylindrical GM or ionization-type detectors, this will usually be "parallel" or "perpendicular" indicating photons traveling either parallel with or perpendicular to the central axis of the detector; for instruments with internal detectors, this should be the angle between the flux field and a specified surface of the instrument);

    13.1.   For detectors with removable shielding, an indication of whether the shielding was in place or removed during the calibration procedure;

    13.2.   Apparent reading from the check source; and

    13.3.   Name of the person who performed the calibration and the date on which the calibration was performed.

    13.4.   The following information will be attached to the instrument as a calibration sticker:

    13.5.   Source used to calibrate the instrument (i.e., Cs-137);

    13.6.   Battery check position;

    13.7.   Relevant correction factors for each scale or decade;

    13.8.   Angle between the radiation flux and the detector during calibration;

    13.9.   Date calibrated the date due;

    13.10. Check source reading.

Procedure for Calibrating Dose Calibrator

Test for the following at the indicated frequency. Consider repair, replacement, or arithmetic correction if the dose calibrator falls outside the suggested tolerances. These recommended tolerances are more restrictive than in the Regulations to ensure that corrective action will be taken before the dose calibrator is outside permissible tolerances.

∴ **Constancy**

Constancy means reproducibility in measuring a constant source over along period. Assay two reference sources, which are obtained commercially as solidified dose calibrator test sources. Use 100-200μCi Cs-137 and 1-2 mCi Co057 in a reproducible geometry for each daily test.

1. Prior to the assay of the first patient dose, assay each reference source using the appropriate instrument setting (i.e., Cs-137 setting for Cs-137).
2. Measure and record background level. Record the results of each test on the standard form.
3. All readings must be within 5% of the predicted activity or the instrument needs to be recalibrated or serviced.
4. Use the Cs-137 source to take a reading on all commonly used radionuclide settings.
5. Constancy testing is also repeated after any repair, adjustment, relocation, or receipt of a new dose calibrator.

6. The action level or tolerance for each recorded measurement at which the individual performing the test will automatically notify the chief technician or authorized user of suspected malfunction of the calibrator are set at 10% of the recorded values. The regulations require repair or replacement if the error exceeds 10 percent.
7. Inspect the instrument on a quarterly basis to ascertain that the measurement chamber liner is in place and that the instrument is zeroed according to the manufacturer's instructions.

∴ **Linearity**

Linearity means that the calibrator is able to indicate the correct activity over the range of use of that calibrator. This test is done at installation and at least quarterly. The range of doses used is the highest patient dose ever to be used at the facility to 30μCi. The initial test or long-hand method requires three days. Linearity testing must be repeated after any repair, adjustment, relocation, or receipt of a new dose calibrator.

Decay Method:

1. Assay the Tc-99m vial in the dose calibrator and subtract background level to obtain net activity in millicuries. Record the date, time and net activity.
2. Repeat step 1 at intervals of 6, 24, 30, 54, 72, and 78 hours after the initial assay; longer if the activity is still not measured less than 30μCi.
3. Using the 30 hour activity measurement as a starting point, calculate the predicted activities at 0, 6, 24, 48, 54, 72, and 78 hours using the following table:

Assay Time (hr)	Correction Factor
0	32
6	16
24	2
30	1
48	0.125
54	0.0625
72	0.00782
78	0.00391

4. Example: If the net activity measured at 30 hours was 15.625 mCi, the predicted activity for 6 hours would be 15.625 mCi x 16 = 250 mCi. If actual measurement times differ from those that are suggested by more than 5 minutes, corrections should be made using Tc-99m decay charts.
5. Once the lowest limit has been reached, a computerized graph of the plotted results is to be made. On review of the assays and the graph, a deviation of ±5% calls for repair or adjustment of the dose calibrator.

6. To create a graph, on a sheet of log-log graph paper label the vertical axis in actual millicuries as recorded on the dose calibrator. Label the logarithmic horizontal axis in millicuries as calculated for decay. Plot the actual readings in millicuries against the calculated readings in millicuries. The actual readings versus the calculated activity must be within 5%. At the top of the graph, note the date, manufacturer, model number, and serial number of the dose calibrator. Then plot the data.

7. Draw a "best fit" straight line through the data points. For the point farthest from the line, calculate its deviation from the value on the line.

Deviation = (activity observed – activity value from "best fit" line)
Activity value from "best fit" line

8. If the worst deviation is more than $\forall 0.05$, the dose calibrator should be repaired or adjusted. If this cannot be done, it will be necessary to make a correction table or graph that will allow you to convert from activity indicated by the dose calibrator to "true activity".

9. Put a sticker on the dose calibrator that states when the next linearity test is due.

Shield Method:

A set of Cali-check tubes may be used to perform quarterly linearity as follows:

1. Assay the Tc-99m syringe or vial in the dose calibrator, and subtract background to obtain the net activity in millicuries. Record the net activity.
2. Steps 3 through 5 below must be completed within 6 minutes.
3. Put the base and sleeve 1 in the dose calibrator with the vial. Record the sleeve number and indicated activity.
4. Remove sleeve 1 and put in sleeve 2. Record the sleeve number and indicated activity.
5. Continue for all sleeves.
6. Plot the data using the equivalent decay time associated with each sleeve.
7. Draw a "best fit" straight line through the data points. For the point farthest from the line, calculate its deviation from the value on the line.
8. Deviation = (activity observed – activity value from "best fit" line)
                            Activity value from "best fit" line
9. If the worst deviation is more than 0.05, the dose calibrator should be repaired or adjusted.
10. Put a sticker on the dose calibrator that says when the next linearity test is due.

Geometry

Geometry independence means that the indicated activity does not change with volume or configuration. This test should be done using a syringe that is normally used for injections. Licensees who use generators and radiopharmaceutical kits should also do the test using a vial similar in size, shape, and construction to the radiopharmaceutical kit vials normally used. The following test assumes injections are done with 3-cc plastic syringes and that radiopharmaceutical kits are made in 30-cc glass vials, If you do not use these, change the procedure so that your syringes and vials are tested throughout the range of volumes commonly used.

The extent of geometrical variation should be determined for commonly used radionuclides so that correction factors can be used if variations are + 5%. A 30 cc vial containing 10 to 20 mCi in a very small volume such as 1 ml should be used. Geometric variation tests are to be repeated when receipt of a new calibrator, repair, adjustment, or relocation.

1. For each step, assay the vial at the appropriate instrument setting and subtract background to obtain net activity. Record.
2. In a small beaker or vial, mix 2 cc of a solution of Tc-99m with an activity concentration between 1 and 10 mCi/ml. Set out a second small beaker or vial with non-radioactive saline. You may also use tap water.
3. Draw 0.5 cc of the Tc-99m solution into the syringe and assay it. Record the volume and millicuries.
4. Remove the syringe from the calibrator, draw an additional 0.5 cc of non-radioactive saline or tape water, and assay again. Record the volume and millicuries indicated.
5. Repeat the process until you have assayed a 2.0 cc volume.
6. Select as a standard the volume closest to that normally used for injections. For all the other volumes, divide the standard millicuries by the millicuries indicated for each volume. The quotient is a volume correction factor.
7. If any correction factors are greater than 1.05 or less than 0.95, or if any data points lie outside the 5 percent error lines, it will be necessary to make a correction table or graph that will allow you to convert from "indicated activity" to "true activity". If this is necessary, be sure to label the table or graph "syringe geometry dependence", and note the date of the test and the model number and serial number of the calibrator.
8. To test the geometry dependence for a 30-cc glass vial, draw 1.0 cc of the Tc-99m solution into syringe and then inject it into the vial. Assay the vial. Record the volume and millicuries indicated.
9. Remove the vial from the calibrator and, using a clean syringe, inject 2.0 cc of non-radioactive saline or tap water, and assay again. After each addition, shake gently and assay as before. Record the volume and millicuries indicated.

10. Repeat the process until you have assayed a 19.0 cc volume. The entire process must be completed within 10 minutes.
11. Select as a standard the volume closest to that normally used for mixing radiopharmaceutical kits. For all the other volumes, divide the standard millicuries by the millicuries indicated for each volume. The quotient is a volume correction factor.
12. If any correction factors are greater than 1.05 or less than 0.95 or if any data points lie outside the 5 percent error lines, it will be necessary to make a correction table or graph that will allow you to convert from "indicated activity" to "true activity". If this is necessary, be sure to label the table or graph "vial geometry dependence", and note the date of the test and the model number and serial number of the calibrator.
13. The true activity of a sample is calculated by:
    True activity = measured activity x correction factor
    (where the correction factor used is for the same volume and geometrical configuration as the sample measured)

Accuracy of Dose Calibrator:

Accuracy means that, for a given calibrated reference source, the indicated millicuries value is equal to the millicuries value determined by the National Institute of Standards and Technology (NIST) or by the supplier who has compared that source to a source that was calibrated by the NBS. This test is to be done quarterly or after receipt of a new dose calibrator, adjustment, relocation, or repair.

1. This procedure is performed using two calibrated references sources Co-57 and Cs 137. The must be 15 microcuries each, minimum.
2. Assay the calibrated reference source at the appropriate setting and record the reading. Repeat three times.
3. Determine the average of the three readings for each reference source. The mean value should be within + 5% of the certified activity of the reference sources, mathematically corrected for decay.
4. Put a sticker on the dose calibrator that says when the next accuracy test is due.

INSERT METER CALIBRATION CERTIFICATE

NOTES

NUCLEAR MEDICINE
B3.3.2   Crash Cart Med Checklist

REQUIRED DRUGS FOR CRASH CART
- ☐ Sublingual nitroglycerin
- ☐ Intravenous fluids (Normal saline (0.9%)
- ☐ D5W
- ☐ Aminophylline
- ☐ Atropine
- ☐ Epinephrine
- ☐ Metoprolol
- ☐ Lidocaine
- ☐ Diltiazem
- ☐ Adenocard
- ☐ Albuterol/Nebulizer
- ☐ _____
- ☐ _____

OPTIONAL DRUGS:
- ☐ Fuosemide
- ☐ IV Nitroglycerin
- ☐ Heparin
- ☐ Aspirin
- ☐ _____
- ☐ _____

REQUIRED EQUIPMENT FOR CRASH CART
- ☐ Oxygen Tank and Regulator
- ☐ Nasal cannula and extension tubing
- ☐ Mouth piece
- ☐ Ambu-bag
- ☐ Defibrillator
- ☐ Portable ECG monitor
- ☐ _____
- ☐ _____

OPTIONAL: SUCTION MACHINE/TUBING
- ☐ _____
- ☐ _____

NOTES

NUCLEAR MEDICINE
B3.3.2   Daily Crash Cart Review
Month of _____

DATE	DEFIB. CHECK	DRUGS STOCKED	02 SUPPLIES	DRUG EXP. DATES (MONTHLY)	INITIAL
1					
2					
3					
4					
5					
6					
7					
8					
9					
10					
11					
12					
13					
14					
15					
16					
17					
18					
19					
20					
21					
22					
23					
24					
25					
26					
27					
28					
29					
30					
31					

Accepted by: _____ (Initials) Date _____   .

NOTES

NUCLEAR MEDICINE

SECTION B4. RADIATION SAFETY AND RADIOACTIVE MATERIALS

B4.1 Safe Use and Handling of RAM Protocol

PROCEDURE:

All staff in the facility that handles or is exposed to RAM, is required both upon hire and annually thereafter to participate in the Radiation Safety Training Program.

The appropriate form entitled "Notice to Employees" must be posted for employee review.

Individuals should familiarize themselves with these provisions for their own protection and that of co-workers.

Instruction of patients, family members and, as needed, hospital staff (e.g. nursing personnel) regarding radiation precautions for all therapeutic procedures and/or when appropriate for diagnostic procedures.

This poster specifies.
☐ Your Employer's Responsibility
☐ Your Responsibility as a Worker
☐ What is covered by these Regulations
☐ Reports on Your Radiation Exposure History
☐ Inspections

NOTES

MEMORANDUM

NUCLEAR MEDICINE

B4.1.1 Annual Radiation Safety Officer Review of Radiation Safety Program Memorandum

Date: _____

TO: _____

From: _____
RADIATION SAFETY OFFICER

CC: _____

Complete Section A or B

A

I have performed a review of the *Radiation Safety Program* and find it to be accurate and complete

_____
Radiation Safety Officer   Date

_____
Radiation Safety Officer   Date

_____
Radiation Safety Officer   Date

B

I have performed review of the *Radiation Safety Program* and am instituting the following changes:

_____
_____
_____

_____
Radiation Safety Officer   Date

Accepted by: _____ (Initials) Date_____

NOTES

NUCLEAR MEDICINE
B4.1.1   Radiation Safety Officer Meeting Minutes

DATE: _____

Address: _____

                _____

                _____

Telephone: _____   FAX: _____

Minutes for Radiation Safety Officer Meeting

TOPIC I

Radiation Dosimetry report: All readings were within normal limits as per
_____ Nuclear Medical Technologist, which is _____ mrem. for the year thus
putting him at Level II.

TOPIC II
Education: Radiation Safety Officer met with all nursing personnel. Radiation Safety Guidelines
were discussed and the topic of ALARA was introduced and implemented.

TOPIC II

_____

_____

_____

_____

_____
Radiation Safety Officer

Copy: Nuclear Medicine Technologist

Accepted by: _____ *(Initials) Date*_____   .

NOTES

NUCLEAR MEDICINE

B4.1.2   Delegation of Radiation Safety Officer Authority

POLICY:
Radiation Safety Officer Delegation of Authority

PROCEDURE:
Delegation of authority:_____
is appointed radiation safety officer and is responsible for ensuring the safe use of radiation. The Radiation Safety Officer (RSO) is responsible for managing the radiation safety program to include radiation safety training both upon hire and annually thereafter; identifying radiation safety problems; initiating, recommending, or providing corrective actions; verifying implementation of corrective actions; and ensuring compliance with regulations.

The radiation safety office is hereby delegated the authority to meet those responsibilities:
1. Ensure that licensed material will be used safely. This includes review, as necessary of training programs, equipment, facility, supplies, and procedures;
2. Ensure that licensed material is used in compliance with the State and Federal Radiation Regulations and the institutional license;
3. Ensure that the use of licensed material is consistent with the ALARA philosophy and program;
4. Establish a table of investigational levels for individual occupational radiation exposures; and
5. Identify program problems and solutions.
6. Review the training and experience of the proposed authorized users, and the authorized medical physicist to determine that their qualifications are sufficient to enable the individuals to perform their duties safely and are in accordance with the regulations and the license;
7. Review on the basis of safety and approve or deny, consistent with the limitations of the regulations, the license, and the ALARA philosophy, all requests for authorization to use radioactive material within the institution;
8. Prescribe special conditions that will be required during a proposed method of use of radioactive material such as requirements for bioassay, physical examinations of users, and special monitoring procedures;
9. Review quarterly the occupational radiation exposure records of all personnel, giving attention to individuals or groups of workers whose occupational exposure appears excessive;
10. Establish a program to ensure that all persons whose duties may require them to work in or frequent areas where radioactive materials are used (e.g., nursing, security, housekeeping, physical plant) are appropriately instructed as required.

11. Review at least annually the entire radiation safety program to determine that all activities are being conducted safely, in accordance with radiation regulations and the conditions of the license, and consistent with the ALARA program and philosophy. The review must include an examination of records, reports from the Radiation Safety Officer, results of the Department's inspections, written safety procedures, and the adequacy of the management control system;

12. Recommend remedial action to correct any deficiencies identified in the radiation safety program;

13. Maintain written minutes of all Committee meetings, including members in attendance and members absent, discussions, actions, recommendations, decisions, and numerical results of all votes taken; and

14. Ensure that the radioactive material license is amended if required prior to any changes in facilities, equipment, policies, procedures, and personnel.

MEMORANDUM

NUCLEAR MEDICINE

  B4.1.2   Delegation of Radiation Safety Officer Authority Memorandum

To: ALL PERSONNEL

From: _____

CC: _____

Subject: *Delegation of Authority*

Date: _____

_____has been appointed

Radiation Safety Officer and is responsible for ensuring the safe use of radiation.

Radiation Safety Officer is responsible for managing the radiation safety program; identifying radiation safety problems; initiating, recommending, or providing corrective actions; verifying implementation of corrective actions; and ensuring compliance with regulations.

Radiation Safety Officer is hereby delegated the authority necessary to meet those responsibilities.

Radiation Safety Officer is also responsible for assisting the Radiation Safety Committee in the performance of its duties and serving as its secretary.

Signed:

_____/_____
                                                                    DATE

NOTES

NUCLEAR MEDICINE

B4.1.3   Authorization of Nuclear Medical Technologist to Handle RAM

_____ delegates the following authority:

Radiation Safety Officer/ Authorized User

To _____
                Nuclear Medical Technologist

under the supervision of a Principle User, with a written directive, the administration to patients of radiopharmaceuticals.

Signed:

_____
Radiation Safety Officer/ Authorized User   _____ Date

NUCLEAR MEDICINE
B4.1.3   Designation of Who May Handle RAM

PURPOSE:
Designation of Who May Handle RAM

PROCEDURE:
The following is a list of properly trained personnel designated to handle radioactive material under the supervision of the listed Authorized Users:

AUTHORIZED USERS:	
Name	**Hire Date**
NUCLEAR MEDICINE TECHNOLOGISTS:	
OTHER TRAINED PERSONNEL:	

Accepted by: _____ (Initials) Date_____   .

NUCLEAR MEDICINE
SECTION B4.   B4.3.1 RADIATION SAFETY PERSONNEL PROTOCOL
B4.3.1   Safe Use and Handling of RAM Protocol

PURPOSE:
To establish a procedure for the safe use of radiopharmaceuticals.

Personnel will be instructed:
1. Before assuming duties with, or near, radioactive materials as part of the orientation program for new employees.
2. During annual refresher training.
3. Whenever there is a significant change in duties, regulations, or the terms of the license.

Instruction for individuals in attendance will include the following subjects:
1. Applicable regulations and license conditions
2. Importance of ALARA
3. Areas where radioactive material is used or stored
4. Potential hazards associated with radioactive material in each area where the employees will work
5. Appropriate radiation safety procedures
6. Licensee's in-hours work rules
7. Individuals' obligation to report unsafe conditions to the Radiation Safety Officer
8. Appropriate response to emergencies or unsafe conditions
9. Worker's right to be informed of occupational radiation exposure and bioassay results
10. Locations of license posted or available notices, copies of pertinent and applicable correspondence
11. Question and answer review.

PROCEDURE:
1. Wear laboratory coats or other protective clothing at all times in areas where radioactive materials are used.
2. Wear disposable gloves at all times while handling radioactive materials.
3. After each procedure or before leaving the area, monitor your hands for contamination in a low-background area with either a crystal probe or camera.
4. Use syringe shields for routine preparation of multi-dose vials and administration of radiopharmaceuticals to patients, except in those circumstances in which their use is contraindicated (e.g., recessed veins, infants). In these exceptional cases, consider the use of other protective methods such as remote delivery of the dose (e.g., through use of a butterfly valve).

5. Do not eat, drink, smoke, or apply cosmetics in any area where radioactive material is stored or used.

6. Do not store food, drink, or personal effects in areas where radioactive material is stored or used.

7. Wear personnel monitoring devices at all times while in areas where radioactive materials are used or stored. These devices should be worn as prescribed by the Radiation Safety Officer. When not being worn to monitor occupational exposures, personnel monitoring devices should be stored in the work place in a designated low-background area.

8. Wear a finger exposure monitor during the elution of generators; during the preparation, assay, and injection of radiopharmaceuticals; and when holding patients during procedures.

9. Dispose of radioactive waste only in designated, labeled, and properly shielded receptacles.

10. Never pipette by mouth.

11. Wipe-test radioactive material storage, preparation, and administration areas weekly for contamination. If necessary, decontaminate or secure the area for decay.

12. With a radiation detection survey meter, survey the generator storage, kit preparation, and injection areas daily for contamination. If necessary, decontaminate or secure the area for decay as appropriate.

13. Confine radioactive solutions in shielded containers that are clearly labeled. Radiopharmaceutical multidose diagnostic vials and therapy vials should be labeled with the isotope, the name of the compound, and the date and time of receipt or preparation. A log book should be used to record the preceding information and total prepared activity, specific activity as mCi/cc at a specified time, total volume prepared, total volume remaining, the measured activity of each patient dosage, and any other appropriate information. Syringes and unit dosages should be labeled with the radiopharmaceutical name or abbreviation, type of study, or the patient's name.

14. Assay each patient dosage in the dose calibrator before administering it. Do not use a dosage if it is more than 10 percent off from the prescribed dosage, except for prescribed dosages of less than 10 microcuries. When measuring the dosage, you need not consider the radioactivity that adheres to the syringe wall or remains in the needle. Check the patient's name and identification number and the prescribed radionuclide, chemical form, and dosage before administering.

15. Always keep flood sources, syringes, waste, and other radioactive material in shielded containers.

16. Because even sources with small amounts of radioactivity exhibit a high dose rate on contact, you should use a cart or wheelchair to move flood sources, waste, and other radioactive material.

17. All doses shall be assayed within 30 minutes of administration time.
18. Always use absorbent disposable paper in preparation area.
19. Utilize ALARA principals, apply accordingly.
    - ☐ Time
    - ☐ Distance
    - ☐ Shielding

NUCLEAR MEDICINE
   B4.3.1.1   ALARA

POLICY:
Program for Maintaining Occupational Radiation Exposure at Medical Institutions ALARA

PROCEDURE:
   MANAGEMENT COMMITMENT

1. We, the management of _____ are
    committed to the program described herein for keeping individual and collective doses as
    low as is reasonable achievable (ALARA). In accord with this commitment, we hereby
    designate an administrative organization for radiation safety that will develop the necessary
    written policy, procedures, and instructions to foster the ALARA concept within our
    institution. The organization will include a Radiation Safety Officer (RSO).

2. We will perform a formal annual review of the Radiation Safety Program, including
    ALARA considerations to include reviews of operating procedures, past dose records,
    inspections, and consultations with the Radiation Safety staff and/or outside consultants.

3. Modifications to operating and maintenance procedures, equipment, and facilities will be
    made to reduce exposures. We will seek and demonstrate improvements, consider
    modifications, including those recommended but not implemented, along with rationale for
    non-implementation.

4. In addition to maintaining the dose to individuals as below the limits as is reasonably
    achievable, the sum of the doses received by all exposed individuals will also be
    maintained at the lowest practicable level.

The Radiation Safety Officer will perform a quarterly review of occupational radiation exposure
with particular attention to instances in which the investigational levels in *TABLE I* are exceeded.

RADIATION SAFETY OFFICER DUTIES:

1. Radiation Safety Officer will perform an annual review of the Radiation Safety Program for adherence to ALARA concepts. Reviews of specific methods of use must also be conducted upon hire.
2. Radiation Safety Officer will review at least quarterly the external radiation doses of authorized users and personnel to determine that their doses are ALARA in accordance with the provisions of Section F of this Program.
3. Radiation Safety Officer will schedule briefings and educational sessions to inform personnel of ALARA Program efforts.
4. Radiation Safety Officer will ensure that Authorized Users, personnel, and ancillary personnel subject to exposure to radiation will be instructed in The ALARA philosophy, and informed that management and the Radiation Safety Officer is committed to implementing the ALARA concept.
5. Radiation Safety Officer will investigate all known instances of deviation from good ALARA practices and, if possible, will determine the causes. When the cause is know, the Radiation Safety Officer will implement changes in the program to maintain doses ALARA.

AUTHORIZED USERS

1. Authorized User will consult the Radiation Safety Officer during the planning stage before using radioactive materials for new uses.
2. Authorized User will explain the ALARA concept and the need to maintain exposures ALARA to all supervised individuals.
3. Authorized User will ensure that supervised individuals who are subject to occupational radiation exposure are trained and educated in good health physics practices and in maintaining exposures ALARA.

TABLE I Investigational Levels (mRem) Per Quarter			
	Level I	Level II	Annual Limit
1. Whole Body (DDE)	125	375	5,000
2. Lens of the Eye (LDE)	375	1,125	15,000
3. Extremity (SDE-ME)	1,250	3,750	50,000
4. Skin (SDE-WB)	1,250	3,750	50,000
5. Declared Pregnant Women(DPW)	40	150	500 per gestation period

I hereby certify that this institution has implemented the ALARA Program as set forth in the Radiation Safety Manual.

_____

Medical Director

_____ Radiation Safety

Officer   *Accepted by: _____ (Initials) Date_____*

NUCLEAR MEDICINE

B4.3.1.2 Radioactive Materials Signage

PURPOSE:

To establish a procedure for caution signs, warnings and labels.

PROCEDURE:

Appropriate caution signs are required in all areas and on all containers where significant amounts of radiation or radioactive materials may be found. These must bear the three-bladed radioactive caution symbol in magenta, black, or purple on a yellow background.

The specific label to be used depends on the type and degree of hazard present.

COMMONLY USED RADIONUCLIDES VALUES	
Chromium – 51	- 1000 µCi
Cobalt – 57	- 100 µCi
Gallium – 67	- 1000 µCi
Indium – 111	- 100 µCi
Iodine – 125	- 1 µCi
Iodine – 131	- 1 µCi
Molybdenum – 99	- 100 µCi
Phosphorus – 32	- 10 µCi
Strontium – 89	- 10 µCi
Sulfur – 35	- 100 µCi
Technetium – 99m	- 1000 µCi
Thallium – 201	- 1000 µCi
Xenon - 133	- 1000 µCi

Individuals shall, prior to disposal of any uncontaminated empty container to an unrestricted area, remove or deface the radioactive material label or otherwise clearly indicate that the container no longer contains radioactive materials.

Posting Requirements

1. Posting of Radiation Areas.
The licensee or registrant shall post each radiation area with a conspicuous sign or signs bearing the radiation symbol and the words

"CAUTION, RADIATION AREA."

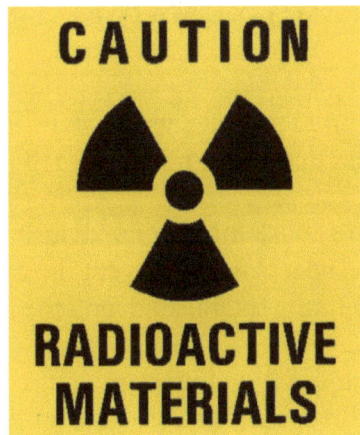

2. Posting of High Radiation Areas.

"CAUTION, HIGH RADIATION AREA"

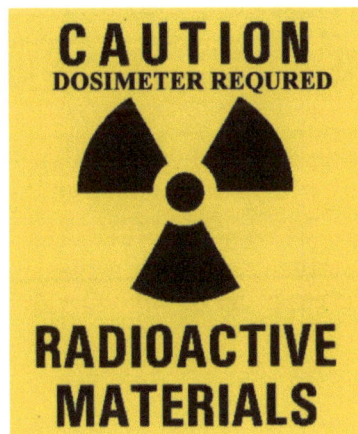

or

3. Posting of Areas or Rooms in which Licensed or Registered Sources of Radiation are Used or Stored.

The licensee or registrant shall post each area or room in which there is used or stored an amount of licensed or registered source of radiation exceeding 10 times the quantity of such source of radiation specified with a conspicuous sign or signs bearing the radiation symbol and the words

"CAUTION, RADIOACTIVE MATERIAL(S)"

"DANGER, RADIOACTIVE MATERIAL(S)"

Exceptions to Posting Requirements

4. A. A licensee or registrant is not required to post caution signs in areas or rooms containing sources of radiation for periods of less than eight hours, if each of the following conditions is met:

4.1. the sources of radiation are constantly attended during these periods by an individual who takes the precautions necessary to prevent the exposure of individuals to sources of radiation in excess of the limits established, and the area or room is subject to the licensee's or registrant's control.

4.2. Rooms or other areas occupied by patients are not required to be posted with caution signs provided that the patient could be released from licensee control

4.3. Rooms or other areas in hospitals that are occupied by patients are not required to be posted with caution signs, provided that:

4.4. a patient being treated with a permanent implant could be released from confinement

4.5. a patient being treated with a therapeutic radiopharmaceutical could be released from confinement

4.6. a room or area is not required to be posted with a caution sign because of the presence of a sealed source, provided that the radiation level at 30 centimeters from the surface of the sealed source container or housing does not exceed 0.05 mSv (0.005 rem) per hour.

4.7. A room or area is not required to be posted with a caution sign because of the presence of radiation machines used solely for diagnosis in the healing arts.

5. Exemptions

5.1. For containers when they are attended by an individual who takes the precautions necessary to prevent the exposure of any individual to radiation or radioactive material in excess of the limits.

Other Posting Requirements

6. Only when there is enough radioactive material in an area to cause a Radiation Area, High Radiation Area, or Very High Radiation Area.

REQUIRED POSTINGS:

Dose Rate	Distance From Source	Posting Required
5mrem in any one hour	30 cm	Caution Radiation Area
100mrem in any one hour	30 cm	Caution High Radiation Area
500rad in any one hour	1 meter	Grave Danger Very High Radiation Area

7. The Radiation Safety Officer will verify all High Radiation Areas and ensure that proper controls are exercised.

Airborne Radioactivity

8. If the activities are suspect to create airborne radioactivity (e.g., vapors, aerosols), the Radiation Safety Officer must conduct the appropriate surveys and calculations to determine if posting the area is required.

9. If necessary, these areas will be posted with a

"Caution – Airborne Radioactivity Area".

10. The consequences of improper posting and labeling Regulatory noncompliance will result during State/NRC inspections.

Notice to Employees

11. The appropriate form entitled "Notice to Employees" must be posted for employee review. This poster specifies:
    11.1. Employer's Responsibility
    11.2. Responsibilities of Personnel
    11.3. Regulation Specifies
    11.4. Reports of Radiation Exposure History
    11.5. Inspections

NUCLEAR MEDICINE

B4.3.1.3   Daily "Spot Checks" for RAM Contamination/Chart

PROCEDURE:

To establish a procedure for detecting radioactive contamination of personnel.

FREQUENCY

Daily, prior to leaving the department

POLICY

Using a survey meter, survey hands, body, feet and clothing, and record the results.
Take a background reading on the 0.1 scale and record the results on the appropriate chart.

ACCEPTABLE LIMITS

No survey reading should be greater than background.
Any reading greater than background will be reported to the Medical Director, Chief Technologist, or Radiation Safety Officer, or their designee immediately.

NUCLEAR MEDICINE

B.3.1.3   DAILY HAND CHECKS

	Jan	Feb	Mar	Apr	May	June	July	Aug	Sept	Oct	Nov	Dec
1												
2												
3												
4												
5												
6												
7												
8												
9												
10												
11												
12												
13												
14												
15												
16												
17												
18												
19												
20												
21												
22												
23												
24												
25												
26												
27												
28												
29												
30												

NOTES

NUCLEAR MEDICINE

B4.3.1.4   Housekeeping Radiation Safety Training

POLICY:

Housekeeping Personnel Annual Radiation Safety Review

PROCEDURE:

1. The Nuclear Medical Scan Room may be cleaned as a normal area.
2. There is no radioactive material kept in this area.
3. All radioactive material and trash are kept in the locked Hot Lab located in the Nuclear Medical Scan Room and must be cleaned by the Nuclear Medicine personnel.
4. No one except Nuclear Medicine personnel is permitted in the Hot Lab.
5. DO NOT REMOVE trash containers posted with "CAUTION RADIOACTIVE MATERIALS".
6. NO sink is to be used under any circumstances which is posted with "CAUTION RADIOACTIVE MATERIALS" signs for any purpose other than disposal of radioactive material. These should not be cleaned by environmental services personnel.
7. Do not clean or touch any article, furniture, glassware, or equipment with "CAUTION RADIOACTIVE MATERIALS" signs attached.
8. Do not remove any article whatsoever with "CAUTION RADIOACTIVE MATERIALS" sign attached.
9. NO eating, drinking, smoking, or applying of cosmetics in rooms posted with "CAUTION RADIOACTIVE MATERIALS" signs.
10. No loitering in rooms posted with "CAUTION RADIOACTIVE MATERIALS" and/or "RADIATION AREA" signs.
11. Personnel who are issued film badges by the Radiation Safety Office should wear them at all times while in rooms posted with "CAUTION RADIATION AREA" signs.

Employee Signature: _____ Date: _____

Print Name: _____

Accepted by: _____ (Initials) Date_____ .

NOTES

NUCLEAR MEDICINE
B4.3.1.4   Employee RAM Orientation-Annual Checklist

INSTRUCTOR:	DATE:
Description of Instruction: _____ _____ _____	

Instruction for the following:
- ☐ State Regulations
- ☐ License Conditions
- ☐ Safety Concerns
- ☐ Record Keeping and Procedures
- ☐ Radiation Safety Manual procedures reviewed and understood.
- ☐ License application, conditions, letters of communication reviewed.
- ☐ Location of State and/or Federal Regulations and how to consult items of importance.
- ☐ Use of Personnel Monitoring devices and limits.
- ☐ Pregnancy policy reviewed and limits.
- ☐ Injection Techniques Reviewed To Include:
- ☐ Measurement in dose calibrator
- ☐ Preparation of skin area for injection
- ☐ Use of syringe shields and rubber gloves
- ☐ Disposal techniques of spent doses and trash
- ☐ Department of Transportation regulations (shipping of radioactive materials)
- ☐ Quality Control procedures for detection equipment
- ☐ Dose Calibrator
- ☐ Survey Instruments
- ☐ Well/Probe counter
- ☐ Gamma Camera
- ☐ Release criteria for patients' breastfeeding injected with radioactive materials
- ☐ Spill procedures for major and minor accidents

PERSONNEL IN ATTENDANCE:

SIGNED	POSITION

Accepted by: _____ (Initials) Date_____

NUCLEAR MEDICINE

B4.3.1.4 Employee Radiation Safety and Radioactive Materials Signs

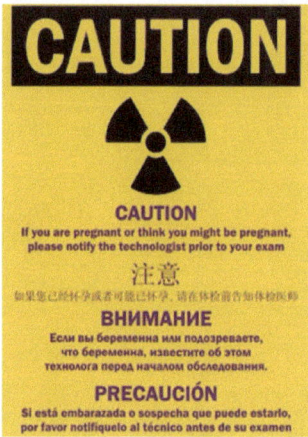

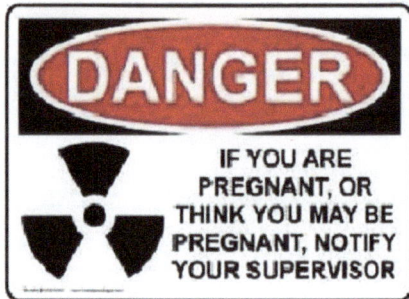

NUCLEAR MEDICINE

B4.3.1.5   Personnel Monitoring Program/Exposure limits

POLICY:

To establish a procedure to monitor all staff for radiation exposure.

PROCEDURE:

1. The Radiation Safety Officer will promptly review all exposure reports monitor personnel or groups of workers whose exposure is unexpectedly high or low.
2. The Radiation Safety Officer will notify in writing any personnel reaching an investigational level of exposure.
   (The investigational level is 125mRems per quarter for the whole body)
3. Individuals who are occupationally exposed to ionizing photon radiation on a regular basis will be issued a film or TLD whole body monitor that will be processed by a contract service on a monthly basis.
4. Individuals who, on a regular basis, handle radioactive material that emits ionizing photons will be issued a film or TLD finger monitor that will be processed by a contract service on a monthly basis.
5. Individuals who are occupationally exposed to radiation on an occasional basis, such as nurses caring for radiopharmaceutical therapy or implant patients will be issued a whole body monitor when caring for such patients.
6. Individuals who are exposed to radiation on an occasional basis but do not work with patients, such as security and delivery personnel, clerical personnel who work in the Nuclear Medicine, including nurses who occasionally care for patients who have received diagnostic dosages will not normally be issued exposure monitors.
7. Personnel designated a monitoring device will be made aware of their annual exposure and have access to the monthly reports.
8. Individuals who handle radioactive material are required to perform daily "spot checks" to check for radioactive contamination of the hands by using the survey meter and recording above background readings.
9. Contaminations will be treated by continuous scrubbing of the hands with Radiacwash in the sink, until a background reading is obtained.
10. All reports from Landauer will be reviewed by the consulting physicist or Radiation Safety Officer and are included in the quarterly report.

Establishment of Investigational Levels of Monitoring Individual Exposures

INVESTIGATIONAL LEVELS (mRems per calendar quarter)		
Organs	Level I	Level II
Whole body; head and trunk; active blood-forming organs; and gonads	125	375
Lens of eyes:	375	1,125
Hands and forearms; feet and ankles	1,250	3,750

Dosimeter processor's reports will be reviewed each quarter by Radiation Safety Officer. The following actions will be taken for the instances in which the investigational levels in the above table are met or exceeded:

Personal dose equal to or greater than Level I, but less than Level II:

1. The Radiation Safety Officer will file a report of the results of individuals whose quarterly exposures equal or exceed Level I.
2. If Level II is not exceeded as well, no specific action is required unless deemed appropriate by the Radiation Safety Officer.

Personal dose equal to or greater than Investigational Level II:

3. The Radiation Safety Officer will investigate in a timely manner, cause(s) of any exposures greater than Level II, and will take action if warranted. A report of the corrective action and copy of the individual's dosimetry record will be kept on file and made available to inspectors to review at the next inspection.
4. Radiation Safety Officer will review the justification for, and must approve or reject all revisions of Investigational Levels.

ANNUAL REGULATORY LIMITS

∴ 5 Rems – Whole Body Exposure, deep Dose Equivalent (DDE)
∴ 50 Rems – Extremities, Shallow Dose Equivalent (SDE)
∴ 15 Rems – Lens of the Eyes, Lens Dose Equivalent (LDE)
∴ 5 Rems – Total Effective Dose Equivalent (TEDE), External = Internal Exposure (Annual Assessment)

ANNUAL INSTITUTIONAL LIMITS:

∴ 10% of Annual Regulatory Limits
∴ 0.5 Rems – Whole Body Exposure
∴ 5 Rems – Extremities
∴ 1.5 Rems – Lens of the Eyes
∴ 0.5 Rems – Total Effective Dose Equivalent

DECLARED PREGNANT WORKER:

∴ 0.5 Rems per gestational period
∴ 0.045 Rems per month

DO'S AND DO NOTS OF DOSIMETRY

DO'S

1. Do wear ring badge under gloves
2. Do store dosimeters in a safe area
3. Do wear the dosimeter issued only to you
4. Do wear dosimeter when working with radiation
5. Do wear the dosimeter where designated (eg: whole body badge on chest area)
6. Do turn in dosimeter to supervisor at end of monitoring period
7. Do notify your supervisor immediately if the dosimeter is lost

DO NOTS

8. Do not wear another person's dosimeter
9. Do not leave dosimeter in extreme temperatures
10. Do not ever expose deliberately
11. Do not willfully damage the dosimeter

NUCLEAR MEDICINE
B4.3.1.5 Missing Dosimeter Form
PROCEDURE:
The following employee's Dosimetry *badge (whole body or ring badge,)* was missing or was unreadable during the period listed below.

Employee:_____ SSN _____

Department: _____ Type of Badge:_____
- ☐ Monthly Whole Body Badge
- ☐ Monthly Collar Badge
- ☐ Monthly Ring Badge
- ☐ Other

Time Period: _____Date of this Report:_____

Please check one of the following to indicate why the Dosimetry badge was not on the Dosimetry badge report.
- ☐ Badge was lost or damaged, badge was not sent for analysis.
- ☐ Badge was sent in late; badge readings will be on a later report.
- ☐ Employee resigned or terminated- did not work during time shown.
- ☐ Date of termination: _____
- ☐ Badge was unreadable by the analysis company.
- ☐ Other explanation. Please describe

_____ What is the Licensee action plan?

_____

_____

Estimated exposure for the above period:
    Average exposure for the past 6 periods (in current calendar year)
        _____ mrem (DDE) whole body
        _____ mrem (SDE) extremity

Employee estimated exposure for period
        _____ mrem (DDE) whole body
            _____ mrem (SDE) extremity
Employee Signature: _____ Date:
Print Name:_____
Radiation Safety Officer Signature: _____ Date:
Print Name:_____
Please send copy to the Dosimetry analysis company to update employee exposure records.

Accepted by: _____ (Initials) Date_____

NOTES

NUCLEAR MEDICINE
B4.3.1.5   Radiation Dosimetry Report

RADIATION DOSIMETRY REPORT

TO: _____

FROM: _____

WEARING PERIOD	RING	WRIST	WEARING PERIOD	WHOLE BODY	SKIN
Jan 15 – Feb 14			---		
Feb 15 - Mar 14			---		
Mar 15 - April 14			Jan 15 - April 14		
April 15 - May 14			---		
May 15 - June 14			---		
June 15 - July 14			April 15 - July 14		
July 15 - August 14			---		
August 15 - Sept 14			---		
Sept 15 - Oct 14			July 15 - Oct 14		
Oct 15 - Nov 14			---		
Nov 15 - Dec 14			---		
Dec 15 – Jan 14			Oct 15 - Jan 14		
TOTAL THIS YEAR					
TOTAL TO DATE					

Accepted by: _____ (Initials) Date_____   .

NOTES

INSERT FILM BADGE REPORTS

NOTES

NUCLEAR MEDICINE
B4.3.1.6   Declaration of Pregnancy for Personnel

POLICY:
It is our responsibility to ensure that the dose to an embryo/fetus, during the entire pregnancy, due to occupational exposure of a declared pregnant worker, does not exceed 0.5 rem. Our policy is to examine your work environment and job responsibilities to assure that you will avoid substantial variation above 0.05 rem each month during your pregnancy.

PROCEDURE:
1. A declared pregnant employee is defined as a pregnant employee who has notified the director or chief technologist in writing.
2. Once a pregnancy becomes known, exposure to the fetus must be no more than 50mR in any month.
3. Pregnant technologists cannot exceed 0.5rem to the embryo/fetus, per nine months of gestation period.
4. A second film badge for waist level reading is provided for the pregnant employee.
5. A uniform monthly exposure rate is encouraged.
6. If the dose to the embryo/fetus is found to have exceeded 0.45rem by the time the woman declares her pregnancy to the licensee, the licensee shall be considered in compliance with the limit of 0.5rem if the additional dose to the embryo/fetus does not exceed 0.05 during the remainder of the pregnancy.

When a worker determines that she is pregnant, she may notify her supervisor and read the
Department of Energy Radiation Dose to the Embryo Fetus
Regulatory Guide Instruction Concerning Prenatal Radiation Exposure,
and sign documentation confirming that she has read and understands these guidelines.

DOSE TO AN EMBRYO/FETUS
1. The licensee or registrant shall ensure that the dose equivalent to the embryo/fetus during the entire pregnancy, due to occupational exposure of a declared pregnant woman, does not exceed 5 mSv (0.5 rem).
2. If by the time the woman declares pregnancy to the licensee or registrant, the dose equivalent to the embryo/fetus has exceeded 4.5 mSv (0.45 rem), the licensee or registrant shall be deemed to be in compliance if the additional dose equivalent to the embryo/fetus does not exceed 0.5 mSv (0.05 rem) during the remainder of the pregnancy.
3. The National Council on Radiation Protection and Measurements recommended in NCRP Report No. 91, "Recommendations on Limits for Exposure to Ionizing Radiation" (June 1, 1987), that no more than 0.5 mSv (0.05 rem) to the embryo/fetus be received in any one month.

NOTES

NUCLEAR MEDICINE
B4.3.1.6   Declaration of Pregnancy for Personnel Form

POLICY:

DECLARATION OF PREGNANCY

Name of Employee: _____

SSN: _____

Date of Conception: _____

The above employee has provided in writing, the Radiation Safety Officer a declaration of pregnancy as of the date shown above.

The NCRP recommendations state that the dose to the fetus from occupational exposure of a declared pregnant worker should not exceed 0.5 rem (5 mSv) over the entire pregnancy and 0.05 rem (0.5 mSv) during any single month of the pregnancy

I understand that my exposure will not be allowed to exceed 500mrem during my entire pregnancy, from occupational exposure to radiation.

I understand that this limit includes exposure I have already received. If my estimated exposure since the above date of conception has already exceeded 450mrem,   I understand that I will be limited to no more than 50mrem for the remainder of my pregnancy.

If I should find that, I am not pregnant, or if my pregnancy is terminated, I will inform my immediate supervisor immediately.

Employee Signature:_____Date:_____
Supervisor Signature:_____ Date:_____

NUCLEAR MEDICINE
B4.3.1.6   Declaration of Pregnancy Receipt

RECEIPT OF DECLARATION OF PREGNANCY

(To Be Completed by Radiation Safety Officer)

As Radiation Safety Officer of _____, I declare that I have received notification from the above named individual that she is pregnant. I am enclosing a copy of the Regulatory Guide "Instruction Concerning Prenatal Radiation Exposure." I have evaluated her prior exposure and established appropriate limits to control the dose to the developing fetus in accordance with limits in 180 NAC 004.13 (10 CFR Part 20.1208). She should avoid substantial exposure variations and try to maintain a uniform monthly exposure (i.e. 50mrem/month).

The dose to the embryo/fetus during the entire pregnancy is limited to: _____mrem

Estimated dose from date of conception to date of declaration is: _____mrem

Remaining dose to embryo/fetus for the remainder
of the pregnancy is: _____mrem

Radiation Safety Officer Signature:_____ Date: _____

NUCLEAR MEDICINE
B4.3.1.9   Radioactive Spill Policy
PROCEDURE:
Policy for and procedure for radioactive spills.

POST IN FULL VIEW

B4.3.1.9 SPILL PROCEDURE

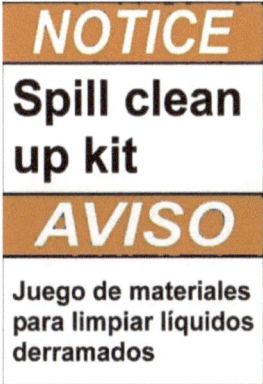

NOTICE
Spill clean up kit
AVISO
Juego de materiales para limpiar líquidos derramados

P-32	10 mCi
Co-57	100 mCi
Ga-67	100 mCi
Tc-99m	100 mCi
In-111	10 mCi
I-123	10 mCi
I-131	1 mCi
Tl-201	100 mCi

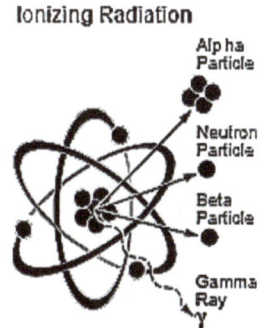

Ionizing Radiation

Alpha Particle
Neutron Particle
Beta Particle
Gamma Ray

TECHNOLOGIST MUST SECURE AREA

1. Clear the area.
2. Notify all persons not involved in spill to vacate the room.
3. Limit the movement of all personnel who may be contaminated.
4. Notify all persons in the area that a spill has occurred.
5. If clothing is contaminated, remove that article of clothing and place in a plastic bag.
6. Notify the Radiation Safety Officer or appropriate individual immediately.
7. Get Spill Kit
8. Prevent the spread of contamination by isolating area and covering spill with absorbent paper.
9. Wearing gloves, disposable lab coat, and booties, clean up the spill with absorbent paper
10. Place absorbent paper and all other contaminated disposable material in appropriately labeled radioactive waste containers.
11. Label container with isotope, survey amount, and date
12. Survey the area or contaminated individual with an appropriate radiation survey instrument, and check for removable contamination
13. Continue to decontaminate the area or individual until decontamination activities no longer result in reductions in removable activity.
14. If necessary, leave absorbent paper labeled "Caution: Radioactive Material" over the area to prevent loosening of any fixed contamination.
15. If necessary, shield the spill area to reduce ambient exposure levels.
16. Wash hands after removing gloves.
17. Check hands and clothing for self-contamination.
18. If individual is contaminated, wear gloves rinse contaminated area with lukewarm water and wash with soap..
19. Report the incident to the radiation safety officer or appropriate supervisory personnel.
20. If personnel contamination is found, the skin dose will be evaluated.
21. After decontamination, if radiation survey exceeds 2mR/hr at 1 inch from spill site or wipe test indicates greater than 2,000dpm/100 sq. cm, notify Radiation Safety Officer and isolate area –test in the Syntrac system (If applicable) for Radiation Safety Officer review reports.
22.

Accepted by: _____ (Initials) Date_____

NUCLEAR MEDICINE
B4.3.1.9   Spill Form

Radioactive Spill

DATE/Time Spill Occurred: _____   ___ **Room/location:**

_____

Isotope: _____   ___ **Estimated**
Amount Spilled: _____   ___
Instrument used for survey of personnel contamination: _____

Personnel Involved:	Initial Reading:	After Decontamination:

Provide a brief description of the accident:

_____
_____
_____
_____
_____

Provide a brief description of the decontamination process:

_____
_____
_____

Name of Person Completing Report:

_____
_____

Date: _____

Accepted by: _____ (Initials) Date_____   .

NUCLEAR MEDICINE
B4.3.1.10 Proper Use of Monitoring Devices/ Survey Meters

PURPOSE:
Use of Radiation Monitoring Devices

PROCEDURE:
Policy for and procedure for the use of radiation monitoring devices.

1. Survey meters will be function-tested with a check source or other dedicated source before use.
2. If the survey meter does not respond properly, radioactive material use must be suspended until replacement is obtained.

Survey meters will be used for all of the following:

1. Area surveys
2. Package check in and out
3. Personnel hand spot checks
4. Any other reason contamination of radioactive material is suspected of possible
5. Periodic surveys of areas such as sinks and dose prep areas will be performed
6. Survey meters must be calibrated at least annually and after servicing. *(Battery changes are not considered "servicing").*
7. A replacement meter must be acquired or use during calibration.
8. Documentation of calibration must be kept on file
9. Along with Proof of replacement survey meter calibration records.

NUCLEAR MEDICINE
B4.3.1.11   Periodic area surveys and Wipe Tests

POLICY:
To establish a procedure for area surveys and wipe tests.

PROCEDURE:

Area Surveys:

1. The survey instrument(s) will be checked for operability prior to each use. This will be accomplished by first checking the battery capability (when applicable), and also by holding the detector against a calibrated check source. If any reading, when utilizing the same check source, is not within +/- 20% of the reading displayed after calibration, the instrument needs to be recalibrated. The reading obtained at each check prior to using will be documented on the appropriate forms.
2. The survey instrument(s) will be calibrated after servicing and at least annually by the manufacturer or any authorized user licensed to perform survey meter calibrations as a service.
3. In radiopharmaceutical preparation and administration areas, surveys are to be done at the end of each day with a low range GM survey meter. They will be recorded in mR/hr in the Syntrac system (If applicable) or on the appropriate form in the Quality Control manual.
4. Areas to be surveyed may be found on the numbered or otherwise labeled drawing of the floor plans.
5. The highest reading for each area is recorded. The Radiation Safety Officer is to be notified immediately of unexpectedly high or low readings. Limits of Acceptability are:
    5.1.   Non-restricted areas: 0.05 mR/hr
    5.2.   Restricted areas: 2.0 mR/hr

If the nuclear medicine lab is ever relocated, surveys will be done in order to evaluate possible radiological hazards that may be present after the old department is vacated.

WIPE TESTS:

1. In radiopharmaceutical preparation and administration areas, a weekly wipe test will be performed.
2. The wipe tests will be performed in all areas noted on the labeled floor plans.
3. These wipes are performed by wiping the surface of the areas to be tested with a cotton-tipped applicator or wipe test smear and the applicator or smear is monitored by using the survey meter.
4. Place the probe of the SM at the surface of the wipe and note reading.
5. Trigger level for notifying the Radiation Safety Officer is 2200 dpm. The Radiation Safety Officer is to be notified immediately of any unexpectedly high readings.

RECORDS:

1. A record of surveys and wipe tests will be kept for three (3) years and included the following information:
   - ☐ The date, area surveyed and/or wiped, and equipment used.
   - ☐ The name or initials of the person who did the survey and/or wipe test.
   - ☐ A drawing of the areas surveyed and wiped.
   - ☐ If excessive readings either are found in the survey or wipe test, the area must be decontaminated immediately and re-surveyed.
2. The Radiation Safety Officer will review and initial these records at least quarterly, but promptly in the cases of excessive readings.

GENERAL:

1. Daily area surveys with the GM meter are to include radiopharmaceutical elution, preparation, and administration.
2. Areas of radiopharmaceutical storage and waste storage will be surveyed weekly.
3. Areas of radiopharmaceutical prep, administration, or storage will be wipe-tested weekly for removable contamination.
4. Surveys for exposure rates (GM's) will be performed with a *Radiation Detection Survey Instrument* able to detect as low as 0.1 mR/hr.
5. Surveys for removable contamination will consist of a series of wipes, which will be assayed using a procedure sensitive to detect 200 dpm.
6. The trigger level for exposure rate surveys will be established by the Radiation Safety Officer in accordance to NRC/State regulations.
7. The trigger levels for removable contamination surveys will be the detection of NRC/State regulations, however, usual action levels for Tc99m is 2200 dpm/100 s Quality Control.
8. Survey results greater than the trigger levels will result in decontamination or shielding procedures necessary to reduce the exposure or contamination levels to ALARA levels on repeat surveys.
9. A record of all surveys will be kept for three (3) years and will contain the information as listed in the facilities license.
10. The Radiation Safety Officer or their designee will review the survey results on a quarterly basis for conformance.
11. The Radiation Safety Officer will be notified of all positive wipe tests and GM surveys (anything over the trigger limits).

Accepted by: _____ (Initials) Date_____ .

NOTES

NUCLEAR MEDICINE
B4.3.1.11 Record of Dose Rate and Contamination Survey Results

Date: _____

Area surveyed_____

Equipment used_____

Serial number_____

Calibration date._____

Measured dose rates in mR/hr or contamination levels in dpm/100 cm2 as appropriate.

_____

Actions taken in the case of excessive dose rates or contamination and follow up survey information.

_____

_____

Survey conducted by: _____

**Areas Surveyed With Contamination And Dose Rate Action Levels
As Established By The RSO.**

Radiation Safety Officer: _____

NOTES

NUCLEAR MEDICINE
B4.3.1.12   Leak Tests of Sealed Sources Protocol

PURPOSE:
Leak Testing of Radioactive Sources

PROCEDURE:
To establish a Procedure for leak testing radioactive sealed sources.

Regulatory Requirements

1. Each sealed source containing radioactive material, other than H-3, with a half-life greater than thirty days and in any form other than gas shall be tested for contamination and/or leakage prior to use or at least quarterly. A sealed source shall not be put into use until tested.

2. Any licensed sealed source is exempt from such leak tests when the source contains 100 microcuries or less of beta and/or gamma-emitting material, or 10 microcuries or less of alpha emitting material.

3. The periodic leak test does not apply to sealed sources that are stored and not being used (except for alpha sources). The sources excepted from this test shall be tested for leakage prior to any use or transfer to another person unless they have been leak tested within six months prior to the date of use or transfer.

4. The test sample shall be taken from the sealed source or from the surfaces of the device in which the sealed source is permanently stored on which one might expect contamination to accumulate. Records of leak test results shall be kept in units of microcuries and maintained for inspection.

5. If the leak test reveals the presence of 0.005 microcuries or more of removable contamination, the Authorized User shall immediately withdraw the sealed source from use and notify the Radiation Safety Officer.

6. Sealed sources containing licensed material shall not be opened.

7. Certain sources approved by the Regulatory Agency and the Radiation Safety Committee may exceed the frequencies indicated.

8. Prepare a separate wipe sample for each source. A cotton swab, injection prep pad, filter paper, or tissue paper is suitable. Number and wipe each source as follows:

     8.1. For small sealed sources, it may be easier to wipe the entire accessible surface area.

     8.2. For larger sealed sources and devices (survey meter calibrator, bone mineral analyzer source), take the wipe near the radiation port and on the activating mechanism.

LEAK TEST ANALYSIS AND REPORTS

☐ Leak test analysis and reports are furnished by the contracted Health Physicist. The equipment used to count samples is sufficiently sensitive to detect 0.005 microcuries of beta and/or gamma-emitting radioactivity.

☐ Certificate of Leak Test must be reviewed and signed by the Radiation Safety Officer.

SEALED SOURCE INVENTORY

☐ A physical inventory of the sealed sources shall be conducted at quarterly intervals:

☐ The inventory record will include the radionuclide, serial number, and estimated activity, the location of each source and the date of the inventory.

☐ The Sealed Source Inventory Report must be reviewed and signed by the Radiation Safety Officer.

RADIONUCLIDE LIST

Nuclide	Half-life	Principal Energies (KeV)	Radionuclide used	Activity (mCi)
C-14	5730 years	B-156		
Co-57	270 days	G 122, 136		
Cr-51	27.7 days	G320		
F-18	110 minutes	B+635, G511		
Ga-67	78.3 hours	G 93, 185 300		
Ho-166	26.8 hours	B-1850, G 80		
I-123	13.2 hours	G 159, 27		
I-125	60 days	G 35		
I-131	8 days	B-606, G 284, 364, 637		
In-111	2.83 days	G 171, 245		
P-32	14.3 days	B-1710		
Sm-153	47 hours	G 103, B-640, 710, 810		
Sr-89	50.5 days	B-1463		
Tc-99m	6.0 hours	G 140		
Tl-201	73.1 hours	G 167		
Xe-133	5.2 days	B-346, G81		
Y-90	64 hours	B-2274		

Legend: B-Beta Emitter B+: Positron Emitter G: Gamma Emitter

NOTES

NUCLEAR MEDICINE
B4.3.1.13 Theft of Loss of RAM

PURPOSE: Policy for the theft, loss, or misuse of radioactive material.

Radiation Safety Officer: _____Phone: _____

The report of
1. Every contamination or suspected contamination of personnel,
2. Every uncontained spill (e.g. Radionuclide spilled onto the floor or not covered with disposable absorbent material or confining tray),
3. Every other misuse such as loss, theft or deliberate misuse of radioactive material must be reported by telephone to the radiation safety officer
4. The Radiation Safety Officer will advise the staff for decontamination, provide final monitoring, and/or investigate as necessary.

PROCEDURE:

Reports of Stolen, Lost, or Missing Licensed or Registered Sources of Radiation
1. Telephone Reports. Each licensee or registrant shall report to the Office of Environmental Compliance by telephone at _____as follows:
    1.1.   Immediately after the occurrence becomes known to the licensee or registrant, of stolen, lost, or missing licensed or registered radioactive material in an aggregate quantity equal to or greater than 1,000 times under such circumstances that it appears to the licensee or registrant that an exposure could result to individuals in unrestricted areas;
    1.2.   Within 30 days after its occurrence becomes known to the licensee or registrant, lost, stolen, or missing licensed or registered radioactive material in an aggregate quantity greater than 10 times the quantity specified that is still missing; or
    1.3.   Immediately after its occurrence becomes known to the registrant, a stolen, lost, or missing radiation machine.

2. Written Reports. Each licensee or registrant required to make a report within 30 days after making the telephone report, make a written report to _____ setting forth the following information:
    ☐ a description of the licensed or registered source of radiation involved, including, for radioactive material, the kind, quantity, and chemical and physical form; and, for radiation machines, the manufacturer, model and serial number, type and maximum energy of radiation emitted;
    ☐ a description of the circumstances under which the loss or theft occurred;
    ☐ a statement of disposition, or probable disposition, of the licensed or registered source of radiation involved;

- ☐ exposures of individuals to radiation, circumstances under which the exposures occurred, and the possible total effective dose equivalent to persons in unrestricted areas;
- ☐ actions that have been taken, or will be taken, to recover the source of radiation; and
- ☐ procedures or measures that have been, or will be, adopted to ensure against a recurrence of the loss or theft of licensed or registered sources of radiation.

Subsequent to filing the written report, the licensee or registrant shall also report to the Office of Environmental Compliance _____additional substantive information on the loss or theft within 30 days after the licensee or registrant learns of such information.
The licensee or registrant shall prepare any report filed with the Office of Environmental Compliance pursuant to this Section so that names of individuals who may have received exposure to radiation are stated in a separate and detachable portion of the report.

Accepted by: _____ *(Initials) Date*_____   .

NUCLEAR MEDICINE
　　　B4.3.1.14　Control of Radiation exposure to Public

PROCEDURE:

In accordance with the regulatory requirements, management and the Radiation Safety Officer is committed to minimizing exposure to Members of the General Public. The following may be necessary as requested by the Radiation Safety Officer:

1. Area Monitoring Badges may be placed in areas frequented by Members of the General Public.
2. Area Monitoring Badge exposures are reviewed on a monthly basis by the Radiation Safety Officer or his/her designee.
3. If these exposures exceed the General Public exposure, additional measures will be taken to assure the General Public's exposure does not exceed 100 mRem per year.
4. Visitor(s) are not allowed in the restricted areas, which are designated by the proper signage, unless dosimeters are worn.
5. Any inadvertent excessive exposure to a Member of the General Public will be addressed with the Radiation Safety Officer and Health Physicist for further action.

General Public Monitoring and Nursing Personnel Monitoring

1. Non-occupational individuals must be monitored when they are required to work in a restricted area.
2. Monitoring is required if the individual is likely to receive an exposure equal to or in excess of 2 millirems in any one hour.
3. Monitoring records should be maintained in the occupational personnel dosimetry records and reviewed, dated and signed by the Radiation Safety Officer.

NOTES

NUCLEAR MEDICINE
B4.3.1.15 Instructions for Family of Released Radiation Patients

Please copy this form to every physician consulted concerning this patient until _____.

Patient: _____ Phone: _____

Address: _____

Next of kin: _____ Phone: _____

_____ was treated on _____

with _____ mCi of _____ in the form of _____.

No special radiation safety precautions are necessary after:_____.

UNTIL THAT TIME:
Persons under 45 years of age should not remain closer than the following distances from the patient, for the time period indicated below:

A- _____ to _____: Permissible distance: _____ feet or more, for _____ hours per week. At other times remain farther than 6 feet.

B- _____ to _____: Permissible distance: _____ feet or more, for _____ hours per week. At other times remain farther than 6 feet.
Note: During the above times, brief periods of closer contact (for example, shaking hands or kissing the patient) are permissible.

SPECIAL PRECAUTIONS:
C- Spouse or other person taking care of patient:
_____

D- Children or pregnant women:_____
_____Sleeping arrangements:
_____
_____

If the patient is to be hospitalized, or if death should occur, notify the following individuals Immediately:

_____ Phone: _____
_____ Phone: _____

NOTES

NUCLEAR MEDICINE
B4.3.1.15 Nuclear Pharmacy Card

SECURITY AND LAW ENFORCEMENT NOTIFICATION

_____ has undergone a Nuclear Medicine procedure involving a small quantity of short-lived radioactive materials. The residual radiation may be detectable externally.

FACILITY NAME _____

ON-CALL PHONE _____

PROCEDURE DATE _____**EXPIRATION DATE** _____

SIGNED _____

TITLE _____

RADIONUCLIDE TYPE AND ACTIVITY

Nuclide	Half-life	Principal Energies (keV)	Radionuclide used	Activity (mCi)
C-14	5730 years	B-156		
Co-57	270 days	G 122, 136		
Cr-51	27.7 days	G320		
F-18	110 minutes	B+635, G511		
Ga-67	78.3 hours	G 93, 185 300		
Ho-166	26.8 hours	B-1850, G 80		
I-123	13.2 hours	G 159, 27		
I-125	60 days	G 35		
I-131	8 days	B-606, G 284, 364, 637		
In-111	2.83 days	G 171, 245		
P-32	14.3 days	B-1710		
Sm-153	47 hours	G 103, B-640, 710, 810		
Sr-89	50.5 days	B-1463		
Tc-99m	6.0 hours	G 140		
Tl-201	73.1 hours	G 167		
Xe-133	5.2 days	B-346, G81		
Y-90	64 hours	B-2274		

Legend: B-Beta Emitter B+: Positron Emitter G: Gamma Emitter

NOTES

NUCLEAR MEDICINE
  B4.3.2   Receipt of Radioactive Materials

DESIGNATION OF SECURED AREA FOR PLACING SHIPMENTS
1. Deliveries of radioactive packages during normal working hours:
   1.1.   The Radiation Safety Officer will advise carriers to deliver radioactive packages directly to the specified area in the hot lab that is either locked or occupied by authorized radiation area workers.
2. Deliveries of radioactive packages before or after working hours
   2.1.   Radioactive packages will be left in the designated LOCKED area in the hot lab by the Nuclear Pharmacy driver where the package will be accepted by an authorized user during working hours.

RECORDING OF RECEIPT OF ALL SHIPMENTS OF RADIONUCLIDES
1. If suppliers includes pressure-sensitive stickers or forms that have the information required you may use these in your records and not duplicate the information.
2. Additional information that is required but is not cued or printed on them must be entered

RECORDS OF UNIT DOSAGE USE
3. For each unit dosage received from a supplier:
   3.1.   Make a record of the Radionuclide; generic name or its abbreviation or trade name
   3.2.   Date of receipt
   3.3.   Supplier
   3.4.   Lot number or control number, if assigned
   3.5.   Activity in millicuries or microcuries as recorded on the unit dosage or packing slip and its associated time
   3.6.   Date of administration or disposal

IF ADMINISTERED
4. Prescribed dosage (unless already recorded in clinical procedure manual),
   4.1.   Measured activity in millicuries or microcuries and date and time of measurement,
   4.2.   Patient name and identification number if one has been assigned;
5. If discarded, the date and method of disposal; and
6. Initials of the individual who made the record.

NUCLEAR MEDICINE

B4.3.2   Survey of shipments of radionuclide, prior to opening,

PURPOSE:

Survey of shipments of radionuclide, prior to opening,

PROCEDURE:

Radiation level limits for the various labeled packages as regulated by the U.S. Department of Transportation (49 CFR 172.403) are included in Radiation Level Limits TABLE.
Most packages received by a diagnostic Nuclear Medicine facility will have a White I or Yellow II label.

Radiation Level Limits by Package Label (U.S. Department of Transportation Regulations)

Label type Package surface limit* 1-meter limit (transport index)*

White	I	0.5 mrem/h 0 mrem/h
Yellow	II	50.0 mrem/h 1 mrem/h
Yellow	III	200.0 mrem/h 10 mrem/h
		*SI conversion: 1 mrem = 0.01 mSv.

1. For compliance Licensed materials must be secured at all times, either by storage in a locked room (such as the hot lab) or by constant surveillance (such as in imaging rooms in which patient dosages may be located).
2. Each order of radioactive material will be authorized (e.g., by the authorized user or a supervised individual).
3. For delivery during normal working hours, carriers will be informed to deliver radioactive packages directly to a specified area (generally the hot lab).
4. For deliveries during off-duty hours, designated individuals will be instructed to accept and secure the "after hours" radioactive packages. These individuals also will be capable of determining whether packages are damaged. If the package is TABLE 9.4 package must be monitored for radioactive contamination and radiation levels. Monitoring must be performed as soon as practical after receipt of the package but no later than 3 hours after package receipt during normal working hours.
5. If received at other times, package must be monitored no later than 3 hours after the start of the next working day.

Each licensee must be able to account for all radioactive materials in their possession. Licensed materials must be tracked from "cradle to grave" to ensure accountability and identify circumstances in which licensed material could be lost, stolen, or misplaced.

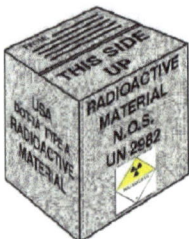

For all packages containing radioactive materials, the following additional procedures for opening packages will be implemented:

1. For packages received under the specific license, the following procedure for opening each package will be followed:
2. Put on gloves to prevent hand contamination.
3. Visually inspect the package for any sign of damage (e.g., wet or crushed). If damage, stop the procedure and notify the Radiation Safety Officer (RSO).
4. Measure the exposure rate from the package at 1 meter and at the package surface. If it is higher than expected, stop and notify the Radiation Safety Officer. (The "transport index" noted on packages with "Yellow II" or "Yellow III labels is the approximate dose rate, in millirem per hour, at 1 meter from the package surface; the surface dose rate for such packages should not exceed 200 millirem per hour. The dose rate from packages with "White I" labels should be less than 0.5 millirem per hour at the package surface.

Note: to convert counts per minute (cpm) to dpm, use the following formula:

$$\frac{cpm}{\text{Efficiency of well counter}}$$

Open the package with the following precautionary steps:

1. Remove the packing slip.
2. Open the outer package following the supplier's instructions, if provided.
3. Open the inner package and verify that the contents agree with the packing slip.
4. Check the integrity of the final source container. Look for broken seals or vials, loss of liquid, condensation, or discoloration of the packing material.
5. If anything is other than expected, stop and notify the Radiation Safety Officer.
6. If there is any reason to suspect contamination, wipe the external surface of the final source container and remove the wipe sample to a low-background area. Assay the wipe sample to determine if there is any removable radioactivity. (The licensee should specify in the procedure manual which instrument, for example, a thin-end-window GM survey meter, a NaI (Tl) crystal and rate meter, a liquid scintillation counter, or a proportional flow counter, should be used for these assays. The detection efficiency must be determined to convert wipe sample counts per minute to disintegrations per minute. Note that a dose calibrator is not sufficiently sensitive for this measurement). Take precautions against the potential spread of contamination.
7. Check the user request to ensure that the material received is the material that was ordered.
8. Monitor the packing material and the empty packages for contamination with a radiation detection survey meter before discarding.
   8.1. If contaminated, treat this material as radioactive waste.
   8.2. If not contaminated, remove or obliterate the radiation labels before discarding in-house trash.
9. Make a record of the receipt.
10. Receipt records must be retained for three years.

NOTES

MEMORANDUM

NUCLEAR MEDICINE

      B4.3.2   **Receipt of Radioactive Materials Memorandum**

To: **Chief of Security**

From: **Radiation Safety Officer**

CC: _____

Subject: Receipt of Package Containing Radioactive Material

Date: _____

_____ shall accept delivery of packages containing radioactive material that arrive during other than normal working hours.

- ☐ Packages should be placed on a cart or wheelchair and taken immediately to the Nuclear Medicine Department, Room _____.

- ☐ Unlock the door, place the package on top of the counter, and relock the door.

- ☐ If the package appears to be damaged, immediately contact one of the individuals identified below and remain with the delivery until it can be determined that neither the driver nor the delivery vehicle is contaminated.

     For additional information please call:

Radiation Safety Officer: _____

Chief of Nuclear Medicine: _____

Chief Nuclear Medicine Technologist: _____

_____   _____

Medical Director   Date

NOTES

NUCLEAR MEDICINE

B4.3.3   Preparation of Radiopharmaceuticals

PURPOSE:
Unit Dose Preparation of Radiopharmaceuticals

PROCEDURE:
To establish a procedure for preparing unit dose radiopharmaceuticals.

1. All Doses are prepared per package insert by the radio pharmacists (Nuclear Pharmacy).
2. After package check in per protocol, each unit dose label is verified for radiopharmaceutical type, calibration time, expiration time, patient name, and amount of radioactivity and then stored behind a lead shield until used.
3. Before administering RAM unit dose to patient, the Nuclear Technologist must visually inspect the syringe for damage, discoloration, or tampering. If uncertain DO NOT USE.
4. The amount of radioactivity is verified by assay in the dose calibrator within 20 minutes of injection.
5. The unit dose is placed in the lead syringe for use to inject the patient.

NOTES

INSERT UNIT DOSE PRESCRIPTION POLICY

NOTES

NUCLEAR MEDICINE

B4.3.4   Administration of Radiopharmaceuticals

PROCEDURE:

INJECTION

Nuclear Medicine technologists authorized to inject radiopharmaceuticals will have written authorization from the Medical Director and/or Authorized User, and will be administered according to the Policy and Procedure manual reviewed and signed by the Medical Director.

1. There will be a designated area in the Nuclear Medicine Department as injection area.
2. The technologist will check label of the radiopharmaceutical for appropriateness for procedure ordered and review patient's medication list for possibility of drug related interactions specifically that may cause performance of the study problems.
3. The technologist will verify the dose is in appropriate range (+/- 10%) by placing syringe with radiopharmaceutical in dose calibrator and adjust setting for radionuclide in use. Reading is entered into the Syntrac system *(If applicable)* or written on injection slip.
4. Procedure should be completed within 20 minutes after calibration time.
5. Prior to administration, technologist will verify written order from requesting physician.
6. Patient identification per
    B2.1.1   Patient Identification Process
7. Ensure correct patient is receiving correct radiopharmaceutical for prescribed study.
8. Female patients assessed for pregnancy and breastfeeding
    B2.1.2   Pregnancy/Breastfeeding Screening Protocol
9. Technologist must verify the
    9.1.   radiopharmaceutical name,
    9.2.   dose,
    9.3.   expiration date/time, and
    9.4.   calibration time before administering to the patient.
10. If a dose is not delivered within 20 minutes of assay, another assay of the dose must be performed.
11. All intravenous radiopharmaceuticals will be given by preparing the patient's injection site with an alcohol swab and the radiopharmaceutical will be injected using aseptic technique.
12. There must be clear documentation of administration of the radiopharmaceutical to include:
    12.1.   substance,
    12.2.   route,
    12.3.   amount,
    12.4.   site,
    12.5.   date/time, and
    12.6.   Identity of the person administering the dose.

13. Syringe shields will be used to reduce radiation exposure to the technologist.
14. The technologist will wait the appropriate time necessary for optimal imaging according to the written policy for procedure.
15. All patients planning to travel soon after nuclear testing must be provided a discharge card with proof of
    15.1. isotope name,
    15.2. dose administered,
    15.3. date/time administered,
    15.4. facility name, and
    15.5. Radiation Safety Officer's contact information.

B.4.3.4.1 Table A Radiation Dose To Patients

RADIOPHARMACEUTICALS SUMMARY SHEET ADULTS ONLY - ICRP publication 53						
Isotope	Special Information	Max. Abs. Dose to Organ		Absorbed Dose to Uterus		Effective Equivalent	Dose
		mGy/MBq	rem/mCi	mGy/MBq	rem/mCi	mSv/MBq	rem/mCi
Chromium-Labeled Erythrocytes		Spleen 1.60R+00	5.92	8.50E-02	0.3145	2.60E.01	0.962
Gallium - Citrate		Bone surfaces 5.90E-01	2.183	7.90E-02	0.2923	1.20E-01	0.444
NaI-123 (oral)	Thyroid blocked {0% uptake}	Bladder wall 9.00E-02	0.333	1.40E-02	0.0518	1.30E-02	0.0481
	0.5% uptake					1.60E-02	0.0592
	1.0% uptake					1.90E-02	0.0703
	2.0% uptake					2.50E-02	0.0925
	5% uptake	Thyroid 6.30E-01	2.331	1.60E-02	0.0592	3.80E-02	0.1406
	15% uptake	Thyroid 1.90E+00	7.03	1.50E-02	0.05550	7.50E-02	0.2775
	25% uptake	Thyroid 3.20E+00	11.84	1.40E-02	0.0518	1.10E-01	0.407
	35% uptake	Thyroid 4.50E+00	16.65	1.40E-02	0.0518	1.50E-01	0.555
	45% uptake	Thyroid 5.70E+00	21.09	1.30E-02	0.0481	1.90E-01	0.703
	55% uptake	7.00E+00	25.9	1.20E-02	0.044	2.30E-01	0.851
		mGy/MBq	rem/mCi	mGy/MBq	rem/mCi	mSy/MBq	rem/mCi
NaI-131 (oral)	0% uptake	Bladder wall 6.10E-01	2.257	5.40E-02	0.1998	7.20E-02	0.2664
	0.5% uptake					3.00E-01	1.11
	1.0% uptake					5.20E-01	1.924
	2.0% uptake					9.70E-01	3.589
	5% uptake	Thyroid 7.20E+01	266.4	5.50E-02	0.2035	2.30E+00	8.51
	15% uptake	Thyroid 2.10E+02	777	5.40E-02	0.1998	6.60E+00	24.42
NaI-131 cont. (oral)	25% uptake	Thyroid 3.60E+02	1332	5.20E-02	0.1924	1.10E+01	40.7
	35% uptake	Thyroid 5.00E+02	1850	5.00E-02	0.185	1.50E+01	55.5
	45% uptake	Thyroid 6.40E+02	2368	4.80E-02	0.1776	1.90E+01	70.3
	55% uptake	Thyroid 7.90E+02	2923	4.60E-02	0.1702	2.40E+01	88.8
I-131 Hippuran		Bladder wall 9.60E-01	3.552	3.50E-02	0.1295	6.60E-02	0.2442
	Abnormal renal function	Bladder wall 6.30E-01	2.331	3.90E-02	0.1443	6.50E-02	0.2405
	Unilateral renal blockage	Kidneys 2.20E+01	81.4	6.20E-02	0.2294	1.50E+00	5.55

RADIOPHARMACEUTICALS SUMMARY SHEET ADULTS ONLY - ICRP publication 53								
		Target organ	mGy/MBq	rem/mCi	mGy/MBq	rem/mCi	mSy/MBq	rem/mCi
111-Indium DTPA (Intrathecal Administration)	Lumbar injection	Spinal cord	9.50E-01	3.515	4.40E-02	0.1628	1.40E-01	0.518
	Cisternal injection	Brain	6.50E-01	2.405	2.90E-02	0.1073	1.20E-01	0.444
			mGy/MBq	rem/mCi	mGy/MBq	rem/mCi	mSy/MBq	rem/mCi
111-Indium labeled White Blood Cells		Spleen	5.50E+00	20.35	1.20E-01	0.444	5.90E-01	2.183
Strontium-89		Bone surfaces	1.70E+01	62.9	7.80E-01	2.886	2.90E+00	10.73
Technetium-labeled Aerosols	Tc-DTPA	Bladder wall	4.70E-02	0.1739	5.90E-03	0.02183	7.00E-03	0.0259
Technetium-labeled Ceretec	Tc-HM-PAO	Kidneys	3.40E-02	0.1258	6.60E-03	0.02442	9.30E-03	0.03441
Technetium-labeled Colloids	Large (100-1000nm) i.e. Sulfur Colloid	Spleen	7.70E-02	0.2849	1.90E-03	0.00703	1.40E-02	0.0518
	Early/intermediate diffuse parenchymal liver disease	Spleen	1.00E-01	0.37	2.40E-03	0.00888	1.40E-02	0.0518
Technetium-labeled Colloids cont.	Intermediate/advanced parenchymal liver disease	Spleen	1.40E-01	0.518	2.80E-03	0.01036	1.70E-02	0.0629
Technetium DMSA		kidneys		0.629	4.60E-03	0.01702	1.60E-02	0.0592
Technetium DTPA		Bladder wall	6.50E-02	0.2405	7.90E-03	0.02923	6.30E-03	0.02331
	Abnormal renal function	Bladder wall	2.20E-02	0.0814	6.30E-03	0.02331	5.30E-03	0.01961
Technetium DTPA (intrathecal administration)	Lumbar injection	Spinal cord	4.60E-02	0.1702	4.50E-03	0.01665	1.10E-02	0.0407
	Cisternal injection	Brain	5.50E-02	0.2035	1.40E-03	0.00518	6.60E-03	0.02442
Tc-labeled Erythrocytes	MUGA/GI bleed	Heart	2.30E-02	0.0851	4.70E-03	0.01739	8.50E-03	0.03145
			mGy/MBq	rem/mCi	mGy/MBq	rem/mCi	mSy/MBq	rem/mCi
Tc Gluconate, Glucoheptonate		Bladder wall	5.60E-02	0.2072	7.70E-03	0.02849	9.00E-03	0.0333
Tc labeded Iminodiacetic Acid Derivatives (IDA)	HIDA,DISIDA,PIPIDA,	Gall bladder wall	1.10E-01	0.407	1.30E-02	0.0481	2.40E-02	0.088
	Parenchymal liver disease	Bladder wall	6.90E-02	0.2553	1.10E-02	0.0407	1.30E-02	0.0481
Tc-labeled MAA	10-150um	Lungs	6.70E-02	0.2479	2.40E-03	0.00888	1.20E-02	0.0444
Tc-labeled MAG3	Normal renal function	Bladder	1.10E-01	0.407	1.20E-02	0.0444	7.30E-03	0.02701
	Abnormal renal function	Bladder	8.30E-02	0.3071	1.00E-02	0.037	6.30E-03	0.02331

NUCLEAR MEDICINE POLICY & PROCEDURES

RADIOPHARMACEUTICALS SUMMARY SHEET ADULTS ONLY - ICRP publication 53							
	Acute unilateral renal blockage	Kidneys 2.00E-01	0.74	7.20E-03	0.02664	1.00E-02	0.037
Pertechnetate		GI:ULI wall 6.20E-02	0.2294	8.10E-03	0.02997	1.30E-02	0.0481
Tc-labeled phosphates and phosphonates	MDP, HMDP	Bone surfaces 6.30E-02	0.2331	6.10E-03	0.02257	8.00E-03	0.0296
	High bone uptake; severely impaired kidney function	Bone surfaces 1.20E-01	0.444	2.90E-03	0.01073	8.20E-03	0.03034
Tc-labeled Sestamibi	Rest	Gall bladder 3.90E-02	0.1443	7.80E-03	0.02886	8.50E-03	0.03145
	Stress	Gall bladder 3.30E-02	0.1221	7.20E-03	0.02664	7.50E-03	0.02775
Tc-labeled White Blood Cells		Spleen 1.50E-01	0.555	3.80E-03	0.01406	1.70E-02	0.0629
		mGy/MBq	rem/mCi	mGy/MBq	rem/mCi	mSy/MBq	rem/mCi
Thallium-201	Male	Testes 5.60E-01	2.072			2.30E-01	0.851
	Female	Kidneys 5.40E-01	1.998	5.00E-02	0.185	2.30E-01	0.851
	Impurities: Thallium 200					3.10E-01	1.147
	Thallium 202					8.00E-01	2.96
Xenon – 133 Gas	Single inhalation with 30 sec. breath hold	Lungs 7.70E-04	0.002849	1.10E-04	0.000407	1.90E-04	0.000703
	Rebreathing for 5 minutes	Lungs 1.10E-04	0.000407	7.40E-04	0.002738	8.00E-04	0.00296
	Rebreathing for 10 minutes	Breast 1.40E-03	0.00518	1.20E-03	0.00444	1.30E-03	0.00481
		Red marrow 1.40E-03	0.00518				

B.4.3.4.1 Table B Addendum to Radiation Dose To Patients

ADDENDUM TO RADIATION DOSE TO PATIENTS FROM RADIOPHARMACEUTICALS SUMMARY SHEET							
Isotope	Special Information	Max. Abs. Dose to Organ		Absorbed Dose to Uterus		Effective Dose Equivalent	
		mGy/MBq	rem/mCi	mGy/MBq	rem/mCi	mSv/MBq	rem/mCi
Tc-99m Tetrofosmin (Myoview)	Stress	Bladder wall 3.32E-02	0.123	7.34E-03	0.027	8.61E-03	0.032
	Rest	Bladder wall 4.86E-02	0.180	8.36E-03	0.031	1.12E-02	0.0414

B.4.3.4.1 Table C Estimated Absorbed Doses to Embryo/Fetus per Unit

ESTIMATED ABSORBED DOSES TO EMBRYO/FETUS PER UNIT ACTIVITY OF RADIOPHARMACEUTICAL ADMINISTERED TO THE MOTHER (MATERNAL CONTRIBUTIONS ONLY)								
	Early		3 Month		6 Month		9 Month	
Radiopharmaceutical	mGy/MBq	rem/mCi	mGy/MBq	rem/mCi	mGy/MBq	rem/mCi	mGy/MBq	rem/mCi
Tc99m Disofenin	1.70E-02	0.0629	1.50E-02	0.0555	1.20E-02	0.0444	6.70E-03	0.0248
Tc99m DMSA	5.10E-03	0.0189	4.70E-03	0.0174	4.00E-03	0.0148	3.40E-03	0.0126
Tc99 DTPA	1.20E-02	0.0444	8.70E-03	0.0322	4.10E-03	0.0152	4.70E-03	0.0174
Tc99 DTPA Aerosol	5.80E-03	0.0215	4.30E-03	0.0159	2.30E-03	0.0085	3.00E-03	0.0111
Tc99m HDP	5.20E-03	0.0192	5.40E-03	0.0200	3.00E-03	0.0111	2.50E-03	0.0093
Tc99m HMPAO	8.70E-03	0.0322	6.70E-03	0.0248	4.80E-03	0.0178	3.60E-03	0.0133
Tc99m MAA	2.80E-03	0.0104	4.00E-03	0.0148	5.00E-03	0.0185	4.00E-03	0.014a
Tc99m MAG3	1.80E-02	0.0666	1.40E-02	0.0518	5.50E-03	0.0204	5.20E-03	0.0192
Tc99m MDP	6.10E-03	0.0226	5.40E-03	0.0200	2.70E-03	0.0100	2.40E-03	0.0089
Tc99m MIBI-rest	1.50E-02	0.0555	1.20E-02	0.0444	8.40E-03	0.0311	5.40E-03	0.0200
Tc99m MIBI-stress	1.20E-02	0.0444	9.50E-03	0.0352	6.90E-03	0.0255	4.40E-03	0.0163
Tc99m Pertechnetate	1.10E-02	0.0407	2.20E-02	0.0814	1.40E-02	0.0518	9.30E-03	0.0344
Tc99m PYP	6.00E-03	0.0222	6.60E-03	0.0244	3.60E-03	0.0133	2.90E-03	0.0107
Tc99m RBC-in vitro	6.80E-03	0.0252	4.70E-03	0.0174	3.40E-03	0.0126	2.80E-03	0.0104
Tc99m RBC-in vivo	6.40E-03	0.0237	4.30E-03	0.0159	3.30E-03	0.0122	2.70E-03	0.0100
Tc99m Sulfur colloid-normal	1.80E-03	0.0067	2.10E-03	0.0078	3.20E-03	0.0118	3.70E-03	0.0137
Tc00m Sulfur Colloid-liver disease	3.20E-03	0.0118	2.50E-03	0.0093	2.80E-03	0.0104	2.80E-03	0.0104
Tc99m Tebrorxime	8.90E-03	0.0329	7.10E-03	0.0263	5.80E-03	0.0215	3.70E-03	0.0137
Tc99m WBC's	3.80E-03	0.0141	2.80E-03	0.0104	2.90E-03	0.0107	2.80E-03	0.0104
F18 FDG	2.70E-02	0.0999	1.70E-02	0.0629	9.40E-03	0.0348	8.10E-03	0.0300
Ga67 Citrate	9.30E-02	0.3441	2.00E-01	0.7400	1.80E-01	0.6660	1.30E-01	0.4810
I-123 Hippuran	3.10E-02	0.1147	2.40E-02	0.0888	8.40E-03	0.0311	7.90E-03	0.0292
I-123 MIBG	1.80E-02	0.0666	1.20E-02	0.0444	6.80E-03	0.0252	6.20E-03	0.0229
I-123 Sodium Iodide	2.00E-02	0.0740	1.40E-02	0.0518	1.10E-02	0.0407	9.80E-03	0.0363
I-131 MIBG	1.10E-01	0.04070	5.40E-02	0.1998	3.80E-02	0.1406	3.50E-02	0.1295
I-131 Sodium Iodide	7.20E-02	0.2664	6.80E-02	0.2516	2.30E-01	0.8510	2.70E-01	0.9990
In-111 WBC's	1.30E-01	0.4810	9.60E-02	0.3552	9.60E-02	0.3552	9.40E-02	0.3478
201-TI	9.70E-02	0.3589	5.80E-02	0.2146	4.70E-02	0.1739	2.70E-02	0.0999
Xe-133, 5 min re-breathing, 5 liter	4.10E-04	0.0015	4.80E-05	0.0002	3.50E-05	0.0001	2.60E-05	0.0001
Xe-133, 5 min re-breathing, 7.5 liter	2.20E-04	0.0008	2.60E-05	0.0001	1.90E-05	0.0001	1.50E-05	0.0001
X-133, 5 min re-breathing, 10 liter	2.50E-04	0.0009	2.90E-05	0.0001	2.10E-05	0.0001	1.60E-05	0.0001

NUCLEAR MEDICINE
B4.3.4.1.1   Radiopharmaceutical Dosage Adjustment

PURPOSE:
Documented system for adjusting radiopharmaceutical dosages
PROCEDURE:

Protocol Must Contain:

1. Documented system for adjusting radiopharmaceutical dosages by weight or
2. appropriate adjustment in imaging acquisition parameters to compensate for patient size/weight.
3. Must be signed by the medical director or a designated authorized user.
4. Before administering a radiopharmaceutical, the authorized user or the physician under the supervision of an authorized user will personally make and date a prescription.
5. If changes are required, they will be recorded in writing in the patient's chart or in another appropriate record, and will be dated and signed.
   Before administering a radiopharmaceutical, the identity of the patient, the radiopharmaceutical, and the dosage will be confirmed by the person administering the radiopharmaceutical to establish agreement with the prescription.
6. Any dose that differs from the prescribed dose by more than ten percent (10%) shall not be administered.

INSERT RADIOPHARMACEUTICAL DOSAGE ADJUSTMENT PROCEDURE

NUCLEAR MEDICINE
B4.3.5   Radioactive Materials Storage and Disposal

PROCEDURE:
There are four commonly used methods of waste disposal:
1. Release To The Environment Through The Sanitary Sewer Or
2. By Evaporative Release; Decay-In-Storage (Decay In Storage);
3. Transfer To A Burial Site Or Back To The Manufacturer' And
4. Release To In-House Waste.

With the exception of the patient excreta and generally licensed in vitro kit exemptions, nothing in these guidelines relieves the licensee from maintaining records of the disposal of licensed material

STORAGE
1. All radiopharmaceuticals will be placed in the appropriate storage area or behind the L-block in the hot lab.
2. Radiopharmaceuticals in unrestricted areas, and not in storage, will be under constant surveillance and immediate control of Nuclear Medicine personnel.
3. Products requiring special storage as indicated in the package insert or the manufacturer's instructions will be stored in a manner to meet those requirements.
4. The licensee will secure sources of radiation from unauthorized access or removal.
5. The door leading to the hot lab will be locked at all times that the technologist or authorized user is not present.
6. Nuclear pharmacy carriers will have access to deliver packages when the technologist is not present.

DISPOSAL OF RADIOACTIVE MATERIAL:
PROCEDURES FOR RELEASE TO IN-HOUSE WASTE:

1. All radioactivity labels must be defaced or removed from containers and packages prior to disposal in in-house waste.
2. If waste is compacted, all labels that are visible in the compacted mass must be defaced or removed.
3. Remind personnel that non-radioactive waste, such as leftover reagents, boxes, and packaging material should not be mixed with radioactive waste.
4. Occasionally monitor all procedures to ensure that radioactive waste is not created unnecessarily.
5. Review all new procedures to ensure that waste is handled in a manner consistent with established procedures.
6. In all cases, consider the entire impact of various available disposal routes.

7. Consider occupational and public exposure to radiation, other hazards associated with the material and routes of disposal (e.g., toxicity, carcinogenicity, pathogenicity, flammability), and expense.
8. The preferred option for waste disposal is to return it to the Nuclear Pharmacy.

WHEN A BIN IS FULL, PERFORM THE FOLLOWING STEPS:

1. Seal the bin with tape and mark with the date, the longest-lived radioisotope in the container, and the initials of the person sealing the container.
2. Swap-out the full bin with the bin in the lower section of the vertical double lead lined sharps, and a new empty bin placed in the upper section.
3. Remove the bin from the lower section of the lead-lined sharps and transfer to the storage area for removal by the Biohazard Service.
4. A lead lined "Decay in Storage" (DIS) area located in the hot lab may also be used for radioactive bins that are full, but that are not yet decayed to a "background" reading.
5. All full bins must be "closed" in the Syntrac system (If applicable), or logged into the decay and disposal section of the Quality Control binder.
6. Short-lived material (with a physical half-life less than 65 days), may be disposed of by the Decay In Storage method.
7. Decay the material for at least 10 half-lives of the longest-lived radioisotope.
8. Before disposing as in-house waste, monitor each container as follows. Record the results in the Syntrac system (If applicable) or Radioactive Waste Disposal Record book.
9. Check to ensure proper operation of the survey meter.
10. Monitor in a low-level (<0.05 mR per hour) area.
11. Remove shielding from the container.
12. Monitor all surfaces of the container.
13. If a container is higher than background, return it to Decay In Storage area for decay.
14. Containers measuring less than background, return it to Decay In Storage area for decay.
15. Be sure no radiation labels are visible.
16. Enter date closed and readings in Syntrac system (If applicable) or disposal section of Quality Control Binder.

RETURNING USED DOSE SYRINGES OR UNUSED DOSES TO THE RADIOPHARMACY:

1. Place all used RAM syringes or unused radiopharmaceuticals in an ammo can provided by the radiopharmacy (Nuclear Pharmacy), and attach a "Secure" cap for proper biohazard protection.
2. Survey, wipe, and log results of the package to be returned per protocol above.
3. Place the package in a designated secure area for pick-up by the Nuclear Pharmacy driver to return to the radiopharmacy.

GENERAL BIOHAZARD PROCEDURES:

1. Biohazard/Hot trash is to be collected, boxed, and disposed of as necessary using gloves.
2. All Sharps boxes should have permanent sealed tops and all red bags should be tied.
3. Label the boxes appropriately for Biohazard Pick-Up and store in the designated area for biohazard disposal/storage.

RADIOACTIVE BIOHAZARD TRASH: SAME AS ABOVE
DISPOSAL OF SEALED SOURCES:

1. Sealed sources that cannot be decayed to background levels must be returned to the manufacturer or a properly licensed radioactive waste disposal facility.
2. Sealed sources must be transported in accordance with the recipient's license and all applicable Department of Transportation regulations.

CONTAINER	RADIONUCLIDE	HALF-LIFE
Short-lived	Tc-99m	6:02 hours
	I-123	13:13 hours
Mid-lived	Y-90	2:67 days
	In-111	2:83 days
	Tl-201	3:04 days
	Ga-67	3:26 days
	I-131	8:04 days
	P-32	14:29 days
Long-lived	Cr-51	27:70 days
	Sr-89	50:55 days
	I-125	60:14 days
	S-35	87:44 day

3. Wastes from in-vitro kits that are generally licensed are exempt from waste disposal regulations.

NOTES

INSERT HOURS OF OPERATION

NOTES

NUCLEAR MEDICINE
SECTION B5.   ADMINISTRATIVE AND OTHER PROTOCOLS
B5.1   Hours of Operation
B5.2   Written Requests for Services

PURPOSE:
Policy for written request for services.

PROCEDURE:
For all procedures performed in the Nuclear Medicine Department, the following program elements are required:
1. A written directive for use
    1.1. This means a licensed, authorized physician must sign and date a written directive prior to administration (e.g. prescriptions).
2. Patient identification by more than one method SEE
    B2.1.1   Patient Identification Process
3. Verification of the written directive prior to administration
4. The individual who administers the radiopharmaceutical must verify the written directive for correct radiopharmaceutical
5. Provide a written record of the administered dose
6. The Medical Director or Authorized User working under the supervision of the Medical Director (e.g. technologist, physicist, or physician) must authorize a written record that documents administered dosage in the Policy & Procedure Manual under the imaging protocols
    6.1. This dose should be documented in the patient's chart and in the Syntrac system (If applicable).
7. Any unintended deviation from the written directive is identified and evaluated.
8. Exceptions to the written directive:
    8.1. If, because of the patient's condition, a delay in order to provide a written revision to an existing written directive would jeopardize the patient's health, an oral revision to an existing written directive will be acceptable, provided that the oral revision is documented immediately in the patient's record and a revised written directive is signed by the authorized user within 48 hours of the oral revision.
    8.2. A written revision to an existing written directive may be made for any diagnostic procedure provided that the revision is dated and signed by an Authorized User prior to the administration of the radiopharmaceutical dosage.

8.3.   If, because of the emergent nature of the patient's condition, a delay in order to provide a written directive would jeopardize the patient's health, an oral directive will be acceptable, provided that the information contained in the oral directive is documented immediately in the patient's record and a written directive is prepared within 24 hours of the oral directive.

8.4.   In NRC states, a written directive is not required for diagnostic tests involving radiopharmaceuticals. In this case, a written order stating the indications for the procedures must be present prior to performing the procedure.

9. Nuclear Medicine request forms must include information about the patient's medical profile, name, age, gender, hospital identification, number, address and telephone number, name, address and telephone, number of the referring physician, clinical background, and clinical data, as well as preliminary diagnosis and any tests required.

10. The Nuclear Medicine physicians should consider the request for consultation, justify and approve the test before it is performed and, if appropriate, modify it after consulting with the referring physician.

11. Request forms should include a space to indicate approval of the test list, the radiopharmaceuticals used, as well as the dosage and route of administration. The form must be signed by the person(s) involved.

12. Patients must sign the correct consent form (if applicable) during the interview and the signature be witnessed.

13. The patient's records should be reviewed and the findings of other imaging modalities verified.

14. Any special technical modification should be written on the request form for the technical staff to review.

NUCLEAR MEDICINE POLICY & PROCEDURES

NUCLEAR MEDICINE
> B5.2   Requests for Services

DATE: _____

Monday through Friday   _____AM   _____PM

Phone _____

For Emergency or After Hours Call _____

PHYSICIAN REQUESTING _____

PATIENT LAST _____ FIRST: _____ MIDDLE: _____

GENDER: M F DOB: _____ SS #: _____ PHONE #: _____

Primary insurance: _____   Policy: _____
Group: _____   Phone: _____
Secondary insurance: _____   Policy: _____
Group: _____   Phone: _____

REASON FOR EXAM:
Abnormal EKG, results: _____ _____
Follow up for recurrent pain after   _____
Chest pain Negative, uninterruptable or equivocal treadmill test _____
Contraindication to exercise Post/perimenopausal female _____
Pre-surgical work-up for: _____
Other _____

201

CHECK ALL THAT APPLY:

- ☐ Angina Dyslipidemia Ischemic heart disease
- ☐ Atherosclerosis Family history Morbidly obese
- ☐ Bundle branch block Heart failure Shortness of breath
- ☐ Diabetic Hypertension Other: _____
- ☐ Previous: cardiac surgery/angioplasty/myocardial infarction/stress echocardiogram/
- ☐ Nuclear study/stress/EKG Other: _____
- ☐ Results _____
- ☐ Other _____

DO NOT COMPLETE BELOW THIS LINE:

Primary insurance: Referral necessary: Yes No   Eligibility verified: Yes No

Pre-cert needed: Yes No   If Yes, ___ on line fax telephone

Secondary insurance: Referral necessary: yes no Eligibility verified: yes no

Pre-cert needed: yes no   If Yes, ___ on line fax telephone

Misys #: _____ Scheduled date/time: _____

              Accepted by: _____ *(Initials) Date*_____   .

NUCLEAR MEDICINE

SECTION B5.   ADMINISTRATIVE AND OTHER PROTOCOLS

B5.3   Duties/Responsibilities of Staff Positions

- **NUCLEAR MEDICINE TECHNOLOGIST**
- **TREADMILL TECHNICIAN**
- **ANCILLARY PERSONNEL**
- **STAFF**

NOTES

NUCLEAR MEDICINE POLICY & PROCEDURES

NUCLEAR MEDICINE TECHNOLOGIST

1. Maintain appropriate records of patient dosages, quality control procedures, patient reports, and other required records
2. Under supervision of an authorized user or Radiation Safety Officer, maintain compliance with local, state and federal regulations in radiation safety practices
3. Review and comply with regulations
4. Maintaining required records
5. Carry out a program to follow regulations regarding therapeutic dosages and follow-up procedures
6. Maintain an adequate volume of medical/surgical supplies, radiopharmaceuticals and film to ensure that a patient procedure can be performed whenever necessary
7. Recommend purchase of protective equipment to meet regulations and
8. Package radioactive material according to regulations and keep accurate records of transfer.
9. Under supervision of an authorized user or Radiation Safety Officer, maintain compliance with local, state and federal regulations in radiation safety practices
10. Perform daily, weekly, monthly and semi-annual Quality Control on all imaging equipment
11. Perform daily, weekly, quarterly and annual Quality Control on all hot lab equipment under the direction of the Radiation Safety Officer or Health Physicist
12. Prepare schedule, dose order and charts for the next day
13. Maintains CE's and BLS according to license and accreditation standards
14. Adhere to Nuclear Regulatory and state guidelines for radiation safety and attends annual review

PREPARES THE PATIENT BY:

15. Verify patient identification, determining pregnancy status, and reviewing written orders for the procedure
16. Obtain a pertinent history and checking for contraindications
17. Ensure that informed consent has been obtained when necessary
18. Explain the procedure to the patient
19. Prep patients to include IV insertion and EKG placement
20. Inject radioisotopes according to exam warranted
21. Perform Nuclear Medicine scans to include acquisition, processing, display, and archiving
22. Participate in stress testing and aid in monitoring of patient
23. Prepare and infuses pharmacologic stress doses such as adenosine, dipyridamole, or dobutamine under the supervision of a physician

QUALIFICATIONS:

24. Successful completion of an accredited training program in Nuclear Medicine Technology. This program shall include training in the basic and medical sciences as they apply to Nuclear Medicine technology and practical experience in performing Nuclear Medicine procedures.

25. An appropriate credential in Nuclear Medicine technology, i.e. certification [Certified Nuclear Medicine Technologist (CNMT) or Registered Technologist (Nuclear) RT(N) credential in the U.S. or Registered Technologist Nuclear Medicine (RTNM) or Medical
26. Radiation Technologist (Nuclear) MRT (N) credential in Canada] and/or state license to practice as a Nuclear Medicine technologist.
27. The technologist must satisfy all state and federal regulations that pertain to the in-vivo and invitro use of radiopharmaceuticals and performance of imaging procedures or Current registration by the American Registry of Radiologic Technologists (ARRT) (N) or equivalent body as recognized by the American College of Radiology, or certification by the Nuclear Medicine Technology Certification Board (NMTCB). and
28. Documented regular participation in continuing education to maintain competence in the workplace.
29. Knowledge of radiation safety and protection, handling of radiopharmaceuticals, all aspects of performing examinations, operation of equipment, handling of medical and radioactive waste, patient safety, and applicable rules and regulations.
30. BCLS certification
31. Effective January 1, 2010, all technical directors must possess either the CNMT, RT (N), RTNM or MRT(N) credential.
    31.1.   Three years of clinical experience in Nuclear Medicine.
    31.2.   Current BLS (Basic Life Support) certification

TREADMILL TECHNICIAN

MUST BE SKILLED IN
1. Appropriate indications for exercise testing
2. Alternative physiological cardiovascular tests
3. Appropriate contraindications, risks, and risk assessment of testing
4. Not limited to Bayes' theorem and sensitivity/specificity,
5. Including concepts of absolute and relative risk)
6. Promptly recognizing and treat complications of exercise testing
7. Cardiopulmonary resuscitation
8. Completion of aha-sponsored course in advanced cardiovascular life support
9. Various exercise protocols and indications for each
10. Basic cardiovascular and exercise physiology
    a. Including hemodynamic response to exercise
11. Cardiac arrhythmias and
12. The ability to recognize and treat serious arrhythmias
13. Cardiovascular drugs and how they can affect exercise performance hemodynamics, and the ECG
14. Effects of age and disease on hemodynamic and ECG responses to exercise
15. Principles and details of exercise testing,
16. Including lead placement and skin preparation
17. End points of exercise testing and indications to terminate exercise testing
18. Additional cognitive skills needed to competently interpret exercise tests
19. Specificity, sensitivity, and diagnostic accuracy of exercise testing in different patient populations
20. How to apply Bayes' theorem to interpret test results
21. Electrocardiography and changes in the ECG that may result from exercise
    b. Hyperventilation,
    c. Ischemia,
    d. Hypertrophy,
    e. Conduction disorders,
    f. Electrolyte disturbances,
    g. Drugs
22. Conditions and circumstances that can cause false-positive, indeterminate, or false-negative test results
23. Prognostic value of exercise testing
24. Alternative or supplementary diagnostic procedures to exercise testing and when they should be used
25. The concept of metabolic equivalent (MET) and estimation of exercise intensity in different modes of exercise

COGNITIVE SKILLS NEEDED TO PERFORM STRESS RADIONUCLIDE CARDIAC IMAGING SUPERVISION OF VASODILATOR OR ADRENERGIC-STIMULATING AGENT STRESS

1. Knowledge of appropriate indications
2. Knowledge of appropriate contraindications
3. Knowledge of advantages and disadvantages of different exercise and pharmacological stress for radionuclide cardiac imaging
4. Knowledge of complications and ability to recognize and appropriately treat complications, including use of adenosine/dipyridamole antagonists such as theophylline and aminophylline
5. Competence in cardiopulmonary resuscitation and successful completion of an AHA-sponsored course in advanced cardiovascular life support and renewal on a regular basis
6. Knowledge of various vasodilator, adrenergic stress protocols
7. Knowledge of the pharmacokinetics of vasodilator and adrenergic drugs
8. Knowledge of basic cardiovascular physiology, including heart rate and blood pressure response to vasodilators and adrenergic-stimulating agents
9. Knowledge of electrocardiography and changes that may occur in response to vasodilators or adrenergic-stimulating agents
10. Knowledge of cardiac arrhythmias and their treatment, including high-grade ventricular arrhythmia and heart block
11. Knowledge of cardiovascular drugs (and other agents, eg, caffeine) and their effects on vasodilator and adrenergic drugs
12. Interpretation and reporting of imaging results
13. Knowledge of clinical use and safe handling of radiopharmaceuticals
14. Knowledge of computer display, systems, standard formats for display of images (SPECT and planar), normalization of images
15. Knowledge of technical sources of error (including motion, attenuation, adjacent/overlap uptake, and reconstruction and count statistic artifacts), ability to recognize such errors and correct them
16. Knowledge of image interpretation, including ventricular size, lung uptake (201Tl imaging), perfusion defect assessment (location, extent, severity, reversibility), noncardiopulmonary findings, and integration of findings into final interpretation
17. Knowledge of gated SPECT display, quality control, and interpretation of regional and global right ventricular and left ventricular function
18. Knowledge of quantitative image analysis
19. Knowledge of coronary anatomy and relation to cardiac images
20. Knowledge of normal global and regional function, the physiological determinants of these characteristics, and the potential pathophysiological causes of ventricular dysfunction

21. Knowledge of reporting systems and ability to generate a coherent, meaningful report that maximizes clinical utility

22. Integration of clinical, stress, and radionuclide cardiac imaging data for final interpretation

23. Knowledge of kinetics of uptake of radionuclide tracers that influence timing of injection and imaging

24. Knowledge of advantages and disadvantages of different perfusion agents

25. Knowledge of physiology of exercise or pharmacological stress that influences timing of stress and injection of radionuclide perfusion agent

26. Knowledge of diagnostic information that stress radionuclide cardiac imaging adds to exercise testing

27. Knowledge of sensitivity/specificity of stress radionuclide cardiac imaging for diagnosis of coronary artery disease

28. Knowledge of improvement in diagnostic accuracy for coronary artery disease compared with exercise testing

29. Knowledge of integration of perfusion and function results

30. Knowledge of relationship of imaging results to presence or absence of myocardial viability

31. Knowledge of prognostic value of stress radionuclide cardiac imaging in ischemic and nonischemic heart diseases

32. Knowledge of impact of extent and severity of perfusion defects and reversibility on prognostic implications of imaging results in ischemic heart disease

33. Knowledge of how to apply Bayes' theorem to test results

34. Knowledge of factors involved with generating pre-imaging probability of coronary artery disease (including age, sex, symptomatology, and stress ECG results)

35. Knowledge of impact of levels of stress, medications, and timing of perfusion agent injection on diagnostic sensitivity/specificity of imaging results

36. Knowledge of improvement in diagnostic and prognostic value with radionuclide cardiac imaging compared with exercise testing

NOTES

NUCLEAR MEDICINE
B5.3   Duties/Responsibilities of Ancillary Personnel

PROCEDURE:

ALL STAFF OF NUCLEAR MEDICINE DEPARTMENT
- Physician's assistants, stress physiologists, trained nurses and EKG techs must be BLS certified *and CVT trained.*
- Physician provides direct supervision; i.e. in the office during stress testing procedures
- Staff directly supervising stress tests are required to be BLS certified with an ACLS trained person on site during stress testing.
- A qualified physician must provide direct supervision (be on site), as well as
- All other ancillary stress testing personnel must be BLS certified

On site means in the same suite or immediately available from an adjacent office.
Direct supervision refers to the persons in the same room as the patient supervising the stress test.

NOTES

NUCLEAR MEDICINE
B5.3   Duties/Responsibilities of Staff (Job Description)

Title	
Department(s)	
Reports to	
Job Description	
Primary Function	
Key Responsibilities	
Minimum Requirements	
Educational And Job Experience Requirements.\	
Abilities Required	
Physical Requirements	

NOTICE: All personnel who may work directly with radioactive materials or regularly visit restricted areas of the Nuclear Medicine Department

☐   License Application, Conditions, Letters Of Communication Reviewed.
☐   Personnel Monitoring Devices And Limits.
☐   Pregnancy Policy Reviewed And Limits.

Disclaimer
The above statements are intended to describe the general nature and level of work being performed by people assigned to this classification. They are not to be construed as an exhaustive list of all responsibilities, duties, and skills required of personnel so classified. All personnel may be required to perform duties outside of their normal responsibilities from time to time, as needed.

HR USE ONLY	
Job code	
Generic title	
Pay grade	
Management? (Yes/No)	
E/NE status	
Last revised	

NOTES

INSERT B5.3 Duties/Responsibilities of Staff (Job Descriptions)

NOTES

NUCLEAR MEDICINE
B5.4   Safety/Security for Staff and Patients

PURPOSE:

To facilitate an emergency response for staff and patients in the event of disaster or other threats.

PROCEDURE

Departments unaffected by Codes should standby for assistance and instruction.
All employees are to be familiar with the evacuation routes and responses.

CODE DESIGNATIONS RECOMMENDATIONS:

CODE ORANGE - Hazardous Materials
            See Section 4. Radiation Safety and Radioactive Materials
4.3.1.13 Radioactive Spill Policy

CODE BLUE	Medical Emergency
CODE BLUE	Cardiac/Respiratory Arrest
CODE RED	Fire
CODE GREY	Severe Weather
CODE BLACK	Bomb
CODE PINK	Infant/Child Abduction
CODE YELLOW	Internal Disaster
CODE ORANGE	Hazardous Materials
CODE WHITE	Security Alert – Violence/Hostage

**For purposes of this protocol, the definition of a weapon is any firearm, knife, or instrument than can cause bodily harm or injury.

The facility reserves the right to inspect the contents of all packages or articles entering or being removed from the facility. Firearms and illegal weapons are prohibited from being on the premises. Weapons, dangerous devices and illegal or unsafe items will be retained by facility management, security personnel, and/or local law enforcement authorities.
Weapons are not permitted on the healthcare facility's property, except for persons who are professionally exempted or authorized by law to carry a weapon in the performance of their duties, such as:
City, county, state, or federal law enforcement officers
Staff contract services companies (i.e., Brinks Armor, Wells Fargo Armor, etc.)

NOTES

Code Blue

MEDICAL EMERGENCY CARDIAC/RESPIRATORY ARREST

PURPOSE
To facilitate the call for the (crash/code cart) and BCS/ACLS personnel to the location of an adult in cardiopulmonary arrest.

PROCEDURE

Dial 911

CODE BLUE

is to be initiated immediately whenever a patient is in cardiac or respiratory arrest. There should be an adult crash cart available.

If a CODE BLUE is called in an area without a crash cart, the designated area will bring the cart.

- **Wheelchairs and walkers should be kept in specific areas to facilitate removal of patients**
- **All staff members are to assist patients in waiting area and treatment areas to closest exit or evacuation route.**

Check restrooms and dressing rooms for patients or staff

Code Red

FIRE

PURPOSE

In the event of a real or suspected fire, the following procedures are to be followed to protect patients, visitors, staff, and property in the event of a real or suspected fire.

PROCEDURE

Dial 911

CODE RED

should be initiated whenever a real or suspected fire is observed.

Indications include:
1. Seeing smoke or fire
2. Smelling smoke or other burning material
3. Feeling unusual heat on a wall, door or other surface
4. Other warning signs as designated by the facility

Code Red alarm may also be triggered by electronic fire detection equipment in the facility

- **Wheelchairs and walkers should be kept in specific areas to facilitate removal of patients**
- **All staff members are to assist patients in waiting area and treatment areas to closest exit or evacuation route.**
- **Check restrooms and dressing rooms for patients or staff**

Code Grey

SEVERE WEATHER

PURPOSE
To provide the procedure to be followed in the event of severe weather.

SUPPORTING INFORMATION
CODE GREY
should be initiated whenever conditions of severe weather are observed.
Staff must prepare for severe weather conditions and initiate individual plans.

SEVERE WEATHER CATEGORIES

- Thunderstorm / Flood Warning Hurricane/Tropical Storm Warning
    o This warning is issued when severe Hurricane or tropical storm is reported or indicated by radar and expected to strike your area
    o Warnings indicate imminent danger to life and property to imminent danger to life.
- Tornado Watch
    o Tornadoes are possible in your area.
- Tornado Warning
    o Tornado has been sighted or indicated by weather radar.
    o If a tornado warning is issued for your area, move to designated area.

PROCEDURE

DESIGNATED ARE A_____

- **Wheelchairs and walkers should be kept in specific areas to facilitate removal of patients**
- **All staff members are to assist patients in waiting area and treatment areas to move to designated area.**
- **Check restrooms and dressing rooms for patients or staff**

Code Black

BOMB THREAT

PURPOSE

To establish a procedure to manage response to ensure safety and security of life, and maintain vital patient care and services in the event of a bomb threat or discovery of a suspicious package.

PROCEDURE

Dial 911

CODE BLACK

should be initiated when there is a bomb threat or suspicious package is found.
The facility may prefer proceed under the direction of the local authority.

Safety procedures take precedence over all other activities except for the provision of immediate medical assistance to patients in life-threatening circumstances.

1. Bombs investigation is an official police function.
2. At no time should the healthcare facility security staff try to touch a bomb or suspected bomb.
3. The role of the facility security staff is to help the police find the bomb, and to evacuate patients, visitors and facility personnel
4. When the police enter the facility, trained personnel will assist in searching for a possible bomb.
5. Security personnel must be familiar with all areas of the building, including closets, restrooms, storage areas, trash bins, hotrooms, exam areas, scan area, etc.
6. Security officers should have keys to these areas.

- Wheelchairs and walkers should be kept in specific areas to facilitate removal of patients
- All staff members are to assist patients in waiting area and treatment areas to closest exit or evacuation route.
- Security officers should check restrooms and dressing rooms for patients or staff.

Code Pink

INFANT/CHILD ABDUCTION

CODE PINK

should be initiated when an infant/child is missing or is suspected to have been kidnapped.

PROCEDURE

Dial 911

1. Secure all exits until authorities arrive
2. Notify Security
3. Check restrooms and dressing rooms
4. Assign personnel to observe parking lot and take note of leaving vehicles

PURPOSE

Establish facility response to an infant/child abduction or removal by unauthorized persons, and to identify the typical physical description and actions demonstrated by someone attempting to kidnap an infant/child from a healthcare facility.

The following information is taken from For Healthcare Professionals: Guidelines on Prevention of and Response to Infant Abductions, published by the National Center for Missing and Exploited Children.

1. The typical abductor profile was developed from an analysis of 187 cases occurring between 1983-1999, National Center for Missing and Exploited Children (Note: There is no guarantee that an infant abductor will fit this description.)
2. Female of "childbearing" age (range now 12-50), often overweight, and generally has no prior criminal record.
3. Most likely compulsive; most often relies on manipulation, lying, and deception.)
4. Frequently indicated that she has lost a baby or is incapable of having one
5. Often married or co-habitating, companion's desire for a child may be the motivation for the abduction
6. Usually lives in the community where the abduction takes place

7. Frequently visits nursery and maternity units initially at more than one healthcare facility prior to the abduction; asks detailed questions about procedures and the maternity floor layout; frequently uses a fire exit stairwell for her escape; and may also move to the home setting

8. Usually plans the abduction, but does not necessarily target a specific infant; frequently seizes on any opportunity present

9. Frequently impersonates a nurse or other allied healthcare personnel

10. Often becomes familiar with healthcare personnel and even with the victim's parents

11. Demonstrates a capability to provide "good" care to the baby once the abduction occurs

12. She will likely remove the newborn as follows: carrying an infant, carrying a bag large enough to hold an infant, covering the infant with her coat/baby blanket, or she may be in a nurse's uniform carrying an infant. The abductor can be a stranger to the child, or a family member, such as a non-custodial parent.

13. A State custody dispute may result in the taking of a child by an official of the Department of Family Services while the child is in the healthcare facility, perhaps for treatment of suspected child abuse.

14. Children can often verbally let someone know when they face a threatening situation. However, some factors, such as domestic situations, state custody, and "wandering" creates a need for an expansion of the infant monitoring system into the Pediatric Unit.

Code Yellow

EMERGENCY

PROCEDURE
    Each healthcare facility is to develop their own guidelines for handling internal disasters in accordance with state and federal law and each department is to develop a departmental-specific disaster plan.
    Departments unaffected by the internal disaster should standby for assistance and instruction.

CODE YELLOW

is to be initiated according to each department's guidelines.
Each healthcare facility is to develop their own guidelines for handling internal disasters in accordance with state and federal law and each department is to develop a departmental-specific disaster plan.
Examples of what might constitute an internal disaster are:

1. Total power outage, utility disruption
2. Plumbing outage and or problems
3. Flooding
4. Explosion without fire

Code White

SECURITY ALERT VIOLENCE/HOSTAGE

PURPOSE

CODE WHITE

is initiated to manage or de-escalate situation of an abusive or combative person who is aggressive, threatening, has a weapon, or has taken hostages within the facility or within its properties. When staff is concerned about their own safety and the safety of others due to abusive or combative behavior, they are to initiate a Code White .
**Approach situation calmly, carefully, and thoughtfully in order to reduce danger to patients, visitors and staff.

PROCEDURE

Dial 911

Combative or abusive behavior can escalate into a more violent episode.
Recognize early warning signs.
No single sign alone should cause concern, but a combination of several of the following signs should be cause for concern and action.

1. Direct or verbal threats of harm
2. Intimidation of others by words and/or action
3. Refusing to follow policies
4. Carrying a weapon or flashing a weapon to test reactions
5. Hypersensitivity or extreme suspiciousness
6. Extreme moral righteousness
7. Inability to take criticism of job performance
8. Holding a grudge, especially against supervisor
9. Frequently verbalizing hope for something to happen to the other person against whom he/she has grudge
10. Expression of extreme frustration/desperation over recent problems
11. Intentional disregard for the safety of others
12. Destruction of property
13. Patients, visitors, or staff at risk of being confronted by a person with a weapon or of being involved in a hostage situation should not attempt to intervene or negotiate.

NUCLEAR MEDICINE
SECTION B 5 ADMINISTRATIVE AND OTHER PROTOCOLS
B5.5   Confidentiality and HIPAA Form

PURPOSE:
Procedures for Maintaining Patient Confidentiality

PROCEDURE:
The privacy rule requires that policies and procedures be established to protect the confidentiality of protected health information about their patients. Personnel of medical facility including Nuclear Medicine will assure that any information regarding a patient's care remains confidential. Patients can expect information related to the care they receive will be handled confidentially by:

1. Preserve personal privacy by utilizing patient gowns, sheets, and changing areas for testing.
2. Keeping exam rooms closed during testing.
3. Serving as the patient advocate by discussing patient's care only with appropriate persons and in appropriate locations.
4. Serving as the patient advocate by involving family members as the patient directs, or as the situation requires if the patient is mentally incompetent.
5. Properly handling all documents and computer information per HIPAA standards.
6. Utilizing appropriate Release of Information forms and Fax Coversheets to external agencies, referring physicians, per HIPAA standards.
7. Provide a notice of their privacy practices to all patients.
8. Limit the use and disclosure of information as required under the rules.
9. Must include a description of all staff that has access to protected information.
    - 9.1.   How protected information will be used.
    - 9.2.   To whom and when it may be disclosed.
10. All employees must sign and date the Confidentiality Statement form upon hire.
11. Personnel must be trained in privacy procedures upon employment and annually thereafter.
12. There should be a designated individual responsible for ensuring that procedures are followed.
13. Any employee who fails to follow the procedures will be disciplined appropriately.

14. In limited circumstances, some disclosures may be made; permitted ones include emergency circumstances identification of the body of a deceased person, or the cause of death public health needs oversight of the health care system judicial and administrative proceedings, limited law enforcement activities, activities related to national defense and security, research that involves limited data or has been approved by an Institutional Review Board or privacy board

The Standards for Privacy of Individually Identifiable Health Information ("Privacy Rule")
establishes, for the first time, a set of national standards for the protection of certain health information. The U.S. Department of Health and Human Services issued the Privacy Rule to implement the requirement of the Health Insurance Portability and Accountability Act of 1996 ("HIPAA").

The Privacy Rule standards address the use and disclosure of individuals' health information—called "Protected Health Information" by organizations subject to the Privacy Rule — called "Covered Entities," as well as standards for individuals' privacy rights to understand and control how their health information is used. Within HHS, the Office for Civil Rights ("OCR") has responsibility for implementing and enforcing the Privacy Rule with respect to voluntary compliance activities and civil money penalties.

A major goal of the Privacy Rule is to assure that individuals' health information is properly protected while allowing the flow of health information needed to provide and promote high quality health care and to protect the public's health and well being.

The Rule strikes a balance that permits important uses of information, while protecting the privacy of people who seek care and healing. Given that the health care marketplace is diverse, the Rule is designed to be flexible and comprehensive to cover the variety of uses and disclosures that need to be addressed.

This is a summary of key elements of the Privacy Rule and not a complete or comprehensive guide to compliance. Entities regulated by the Rule are obligated to comply with all of its applicable requirements and should not rely on this summary as a source of legal information or advice. To make it easier for entities to review the complete requirements of the Rule, provisions of the Rule referenced in this summary are cited in notes at the end of this document.

To view the entire Rule: http://www.hhs.gov/ocr/hipaa.

Protected Health Information.
The Privacy Rule protects all "individually identifiable health information" held or transmitted by a covered entity or its business associate, in any form or media, whether electronic, paper, or oral. The Privacy Rule calls this information "protected health information (PHI)."

NUCLEAR MEDICINE
    B5.5   HIPAA Confidentiality

STATEMENT OF CONFIDENTIALITY

I understand and agree that in the performance of my duties as an employee, I must hold medical information in confidence both inside and outside of the office.

Per HIPAA standards, each employee is required to safeguard any and all medical record(s) against damage, loss, tampering, and unauthorized use. I understand that releasing or misusing medical information may result in termination.

My signature on this document indicates my review and understanding of this policy regarding patient confidentiality.

_____

Employee Signature

Accepted by: _____ (Initials) Date_____

NOTES

NUCLEAR MEDICINE

B5.5   HIPAA Consent to the Use and Disclosure of My Protected Health Information

I understand that _____ creates and maintains medical and related records that include personal healthcare information, including my health history, symptoms, examination and test results, diagnoses, treatment, and any plans for future care or treatment (my "Health Information").

I understand and consent to the use and disclosure of my Health Information by my Provider for the following purposes:

- ☐ My treatment, including the provision, coordination, or management of my healthcare and related services,
- ☐ including the coordination or management of my care and consultation between healthcare providers related to my treatment, or my referral to another healthcare provider.
- ☐ Payment for healthcare services provided to me, including activities undertaken by a health plan to determine coverage or the provision of benefits to me, by my Provider or a health plan to obtain or provide reimbursement for my care, or otherwise related to me.

My Provider's internal operations, including the following:

- ☐ Quality assessment and improvement activities;
- ☐ Reviewing provider performance and training;
- ☐ Activities relating to health insurance and benefits;
- ☐ Conducting or arranging for medical review, legal services, and audits;
- ☐ Business planning and development; and
- ☐ Business management and general administrative activities including customer service, resolution of
- ☐ Internal grievances, due diligence, and creating de-identified healthcare information.

I understand and agree that

- ☐ I have the right to review my Provider's Notice of Privacy Practices for Protected Health Information, which provides a more complete description of information uses and disclosures, prior to signing this Consent.
- ☐ I understand that my Provider may change its Notice of Privacy Practices for Protected Health Information from time to time and that notice of such changes will be posted at front desk.
- ☐ I understand that I have the right to request restrictions as to how my Health Information may be used or disclosed to carry out treatment, payment, or healthcare operations.
- ☐ I understand and agree that my Provider is not required to agree to any restrictions that I may request, but if my Provider agrees, it will be bound by that restriction.
- ☐ I understand that I may revoke this Consent by notifying my Provider in writing that I revoke this Consent unless my Provider has used or disclosed my Health Information in reliance on this Consent.
- ☐ I understand and agree that my Provider has the right to disclose relevant Health Information to my family member, other relative, close personal friend, or anyone identified by me.

_____ _____
Signature of Patient or Legal Representative Please Print Full Name of Patient

_____ _____
Date   Date of Birth/Social Security Number

_____
Signature of Witness

NOTES

NUCLEAR MEDICINE
B5.5 HIPAA FAX COVER

PROTECTED HEALTH INFORMATION

Confidential Health Information Enclosed. Health care information is personal and sensitive. It is being faxed to you after appropriate authorization from the patient or under circumstances that do not require patient authorization. You, the recipient, are obligated to maintain this information in a safe, secure and confidential manner. Re-disclosure without additional patient consent or authorization or as permitted by law is prohibited. Unauthorized re-disclosure or failure to maintain the confidentiality of this information could subject you to penalties under Federal and/or State law.

Date Transmitted: _____ Time Transmitted: _____

Number of Pages (including cover sheet):_____

Intended Recipient: _____

Facility: _____

Address: _____

Telephone #: _____ Fax #: _____

Documents being faxed: Clinic Records

PT_____

_____

Confidentiality Statement:
The information contained in this facsimile transmission is privileged and confidential and is intended only for the use of the recipient listed above. If you are neither the intended recipient or the employee or agent of the intended recipient responsible for the delivery of this information, you are hereby notified that the disclosure, copying, use or distribution of this information is strictly prohibited. If you have received this transmission in error, please notify us immediately by telephone to arrange for the return of the transmitted documents to us or to verify their destruction.

Please contact _____ at _____ to verify receipt of this Fax or to report problems with the transmission.

Verification of Transmission of Particularly Sensitive Health Information:

I verify the receiver of this Fax has confirmed its transmission:
Name:_____ Date:_____ Time:_____

I verify that I have confirmed the receipt of this Fax transmission by phone:
Name:_____ Date:_____ Time:_____

NOTES

NUCLEAR MEDICINE
B5.5   HIPAA CONFIDENTIALITY

STATEMENT OF CONFIDENTIALITY

I understand and agree that in the performance of my duties as an employee, I must hold medical information in confidence both inside and outside of the office.

Per HIPAA standards, each employee is required to safeguard any and all medical record(s) against damage, loss, tampering, and unauthorized use. I understand that releasing or misusing medical information may result in termination.

My signature on this document indicates my review and understanding of this policy regarding patient confidentiality.

_____

Employee Signature

Accepted by: _____ *(Initials) Date*_____

NOTES

NUCLEAR MEDICINE
> ### SECTION B5.   ADMINISTRATIVE AND OTHER PROTOCOLS
> B5.6   Informed Consent and Form

PURPOSE:
Procedures for Obtaining Patient Consent

PROCEDURE:
A patient consent is to provide the patient with the information regarding the test/procedure and to obtain patient approval.
It is the responsibility of the Medical Director, supervising physician, or their designee to obtain the consent prior to the start of the test/procedure. The information shall include an explanation of the procedure; the medical value of the procedure, significant risks, and possible adverse reactions.

If the patient refuses the procedure, the Medical Director, supervising physician, or their designee, will inform the patient of the medical consequences that might occur because of the action.

NOTES

NUCLEAR MEDICINE
      B5.6   Consent for Nuclear Cardiology Testing

PROCEDURE:

I, _____, authorize the physicians of _____, and such assistants as they may designate, to administer and conduct the exercise portion of the nuclear cardiology procedure. This test was designed to measure my fitness for work and/or sport, to determine the presence or absence of clinically significant heart disease, and/or evaluate the effectiveness of my current therapy.

I understand that I will walk on a motor-driven treadmill or be given a pharmaceutical to simulate stress. During the performance of physical or chemical activity, my electrocardiogram and blood pressure will be monitored and recorded at periodic intervals. Exercise will be progressively increased or the pharmaceutical continued, until I attain a predetermined endpoint corresponding to moderate exercise stress or become distressed in any way or develop any abnormal response the physician considers significant, whichever of the above comes first.

Every effort will be made to conduct the test in such a way as to minimize discomfort and risk, however, I understand that this is a cardiac stress test and that just as with other types of diagnostic tests, there are potential risks. These may include episodes of transient lightheadedness, fainting, chest discomfort, leg cramps, and very rarely heart attacks. I further understand that the laboratory is properly equipped for such situations and that its professional personnel are trained to administer the emergency care necessary. As part of this consent form I agree to allow my physician to perform any emergency procedures deemed appropriate during the course of this procedure.

I understand that if I choose not to engage in this test, my physician may be unable to determine an appropriate plan of medical management.

The information obtained from the test will be treated as privileged and confidential, and will not be released or revealed to any person except my physician. The information obtained, however, may be used for statistical or scientific purposes with my right to privacy retained.

For women of childbearing age, between 11-60 years old.

Is there any chance you might be pregnant or breastfeeding: YES   NO
             (please circle one)

This test and form has been explained to me, any questions I had have has been answered, and I voluntarily accept the risks associated with the above procedure.

_____

Patient Signature   Date

_____

Witness Signature   Date

Accepted by: _____ (Initials) Date_____ .

NOTES

NUCLEAR MEDICINE
SECTION B5.   ADMINISTRATIVE AND OTHER PROTOCOLS
B5.8   Infection Control
PROCEDURE:
Infection Control and Standard Precautions

GENERAL GUIDELINES
1. Do not bring purses or other valuables to clinical area.
2. Always wear proper identification
3. Always be aware of your surroundings and alert for any improper activities or individuals.

HAND WASHING IS EXPECTED OF PERSONNEL:
1. Before and after work shift
2. Before and after contact with each patient
3. Before handling food or preparing and administering medications
4. After cleaning equipment or its surfaces.
5. Prior to and after breaks or at mealtime.
6. Before and after eating or smoking
7. After using restroom.
8. After removing gloves.
9. When obviously soiled.
10. After contact with soiled material or equipment
11. After blowing your nose or covering a sneeze
12. Before any contact with your eyes or contact lenses
13. Whenever you think they may be contaminated

HAND WASHING PROCEDURE:
1. Wet hand and wrists with warm water.
2. Apply generous soap.
3. Work into lather and rub to create friction to palms, back of hands, fingers, between fingers, under fingernails, and wrists.
4. Rinse thoroughly starting at the wrists toward fingertips–leave water running.
5. Dry thoroughly with paper towels.
6. Turn faucet off with the paper towel.

STERILE EQUIPMENT AND SINGLE USE ITEMS
To help prevent the spread of infection and prevent cross contamination of sterile equipment and supplies:
1. Items labeled disposable or single use will be discarded after use with each patient.
2. If a sterile seal is broken or sterile package seal is of question, item must either be discarded or returned to the manufacturer.
3. All sterile items will be stored in their original packing container.
4. It is the responsibility of the Technical Director, or their designee, to inspect and replace sterile supplies and equipment for expiration dates on a regular basis.
5. Outdated sterile supplies will not be used for patient care.

PATIENT PROTECTIVE EQUIPMENT

By use of a consistent approach to manage body fluids and substances, the transmission of potentially infectious waste will be eliminated.

1. Treat the blood & body fluids of all people as though they are potentially infectious.
2. A standard precaution focuses on isolating the body substances–blood, feces, urine, wound drainage, oral secretions–with the use of personal protective equipment.
3. The use of such equipment is consistent with the recommendations from the centers for disease control that considers all blood and body fluids as potentially infectious regardless of the patients' diagnosis.
4. Wear gloves when it is likely that the hands will be in contact with body substances such as blood, urine, feces, wound drainage, oral secretions, sputum, and vomitus.
5. Protect clothing with a plastic gown when it is likely that the clothes will be splashed with body substances.
6. Wear a mask and/or eye protection when it is likely that the eyes or mucus membranes have the potential to be contacted.
7. Always wash hands thoroughly after each encounter.
8. Discard uncapped needles/syringe units and sharps in puncture resistant containers for this purpose.

GLOVES

1. All staff are required to wear gloves when in contact with patients
2. To prevent the infection and spread of infection, all staff are required to wear gloves when they have broken skin
3. Disposable gloves are to be worn when contact with blood or body fluid is possible.
4. Disposable gloves are to be worn when an IV or medication is dispensed with a needle.
5. Disposable gloves are to be removed and discarded after *every* patient
6. Disposable gloves are to be disposed of in the appropriate container.

GOWNS

1. Gowns are worn when soiling of clothing is anticipated.
2. Gowns are to be removed after each encounter and disposed in appropriate container.

MASKS
1. Masks are to be worn if aerosolization or splattering of blood or body fluids is possible.
2. Disposable masks are to be worn only once and discarded after each encounter.
3. Masks are not to be lowered around the neck and reused.
4. Masks should cover both the mouth and nose with no gaps.
5. All staff are to wear masks when they have a cold or allergy .

EYE PROTECTION
1. Corrective glasses are *not* a substitute for goggles/face shield.
2. Either goggles or a face shield, are to be worn if aerosolization or splattering of body fluids is anticipated.
3. Eye protections may be reusable if they are cleaned with the proper disinfectant, such as alcohol, after each use.

NEEDLES AND SHARPS CONTAINERS
To prevent the accidental injury from a needle stick and to prevent the possible spread in infection or disease the following procedure will be utilized.

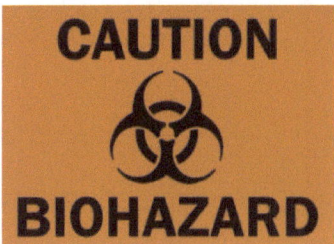

1. Used syringes/needles and disposable surgical "sharps" will be disposed of in the specified puncture resistant container that is red in color with a biohazard symbol.

Sharps are *never* to be placed in the regular trash.
2. Needles should *not* be bent, broken, cut or re-capped prior to disposal.
3. If re-capping is required, then use the one-handed technique.
    3.1. Place needle cap on table
    3.2. Holding the syringe only, guide needle into cap
    3.3. Lift up syringe so cap is sitting on needle hub
    3.4. Secure needle cap into place
4. When the container is near full it should be closed and replaced with a new one. Do not wait until filled to capacity

The used container is to be placed in the proper storage area for pick up.OCCURS:
5. Wash the injured area immediately with warm

1. IF A NEEDLE/SHARP INJURY water and soap.
2. Notify the Technical Director or Medical Director immediately.
3. Arrangements are to be made with the medical personnel for prophylaxis treatment.
4. As indicated, blood will be drawn from the patient to test for HIV/Hepatitis status.
5. Incident report is to be completed.

GENERAL CARE AND CLEANING
1. The environment should be kept clean and uncluttered.
2. There should be no obstacles in the way so as to prevent ease of movement.
3. Equipment and other patient care items must be cleaned between every patient.
4. All linens must be changed between every patient.
5. Countertops, chairs, exam tables, must be cleaned with a disinfectant daily and as needed.
6. Carpeted and tiled areas must be swept and mopped, and restroom facilities cleaned by an environmental services employee daily or as needed throughout the day.
7. Front entrance, sidewalk and parking areas must be kept free of obstacles and trash.
8. During harsh weather, all undertakings must be made to keep the facility safe
9. Outside environment must be kept free of obstacles and trash.

ROUTINE SANITATION
1. All windows will remain closed.
2. Trash must be bagged daily.
3. All bagged trash must be stored in the appropriate containers and placed in the designated areas for pick up.
4. No radioactive waste will be flushed into the sanitation system,–see disposal guidelines in the radiation safety section.

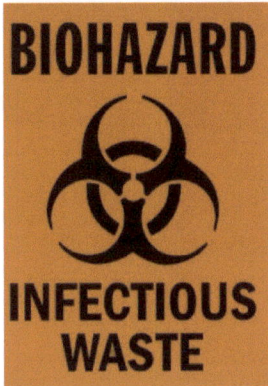

BIOLOGICAL AND BIOHAZARD WASTE

∴ All waste contaminated with body fluids must be placed in closable, leak proof containers that are red/orange in color with the biohazard symbol. These containers are to be placed in the designated storage area for pick up.

LAUNDRY

1. Discard used disposable linens in the regular trash.
1.1. If soiled with body fluids follow the biological waste guidelines.

Non-Disposable Linens

2. Clean linens are placed and stored in the appropriate designated "clean" storage area, or in closed storage areas in each room.
3. Linens are changed between each patient.
4. All patients are given clean gowns.
5. All used linens are to be placed in the appropriate designated container.
6. All linen bags are to be changed daily and placed in the appropriate storage area.

SPECIMENS

Laboratory specimens are to be collected utilizing universal precautions to prevent the contamination of the staff members, work environment, and cross contamination to other patients.

1. Instruct the patient carefully of the procedure.
2. Wash hands.
3. Assemble the needed supplies.
4. Use the appropriate protective equipment (gloves, gown,).
5. Obtain the specimen.
6. Label the specimen.
7. Remove and discard the protective equipment.
8. Place the specimen in a protective sealed container.
9. Place the specimen in the designated area for pick up.

NUCLEAR MEDICINE
OSHA FACT SHEET

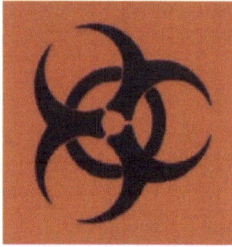

WHAT ARE BLOODBORNE PATHOGENS?

Bloodborne pathogens are infectious materials in blood that can cause disease in humans, including hepatitis B and C and human immunodeficiency virus, or HIV.

Workers exposed to these pathogens risk serious illness or death.

The full text of *OSHA's Bloodborne Pathogens Standard*, published in *Title 29 Code of Federal Regulations 1910.1030*, details what employers must do to protect workers whose jobs put them at a reasonable risk of coming into contact with blood and other potentially infectious materials. The standard requires employers to do the following:

1. Establish an exposure control plan. This is a written plan to eliminate or minimize employee exposures.

    1.1. Employers must update the plan annually to reflect technological changes that will help eliminate or reduce exposure to bloodborne pathogens.

    1.2. In the plan, employers must document annually that they have considered and implemented safer medical devices, if feasible, and that they have solicited input from frontline workers in identifying, evaluating, and selecting engineering controls.

2. Use engineering controls.

    2.1. These are devices that isolate or remove the bloodborne pathogen hazard from the workplace.

    2.2. They include sharps disposal containers, self-sheathing needles, and safer medical devices such as sharps with engineered sharps-injury protection and needleless systems.

3. Enforce work practice controls.

    3.1. These are practices that reduce the likelihood of exposure by changing the way a task is performed.

    3.2. They include appropriate procedures for hand washing, sharps disposing, lab specimen packaging, laundry handling, and contaminated material cleaning.

4. Provide personal protective equipment such as gloves, gowns, and masks.

    4.1. Employers must clean, repair, and replace this equipment as needed.

5. Make available Hepatitis B vaccinations to all personnel with occupational exposure to bloodborne pathogens within 10 days of assignment.

6. Provide post-exposure follow-up to any worker who experiences an exposure incident, at no cost to the worker.

    6.1. This includes conducting laboratory tests; providing confidential medical evaluation, identifying, and testing the source individual, if feasible;

    6.2. testing the exposed employee's blood, if the worker consents;

    6.3. performing post-exposure prophylaxis; offering counseling;

    6.4. and evaluating reported illnesses.

    6.5. All diagnoses must remain confidential.

7. Use labels and signs to communicate hazards.

8. The standard requires warning labels affixed to containers of regulated waste, refrigerators and freezers, and other containers used to store or transplant blood or other potentially infectious materials.

9. Facilities may use red bags or containers instead of labels.

10. Employers also must post signs to identify restricted areas.

PROVIDE INFORMATION AND TRAINING TO PERSONNEL.

11. Employers must ensure that their personnel s receive regular training that covers the dangers of bloodborne pathogens, preventive practices, and post-exposure procedures.

12. Employers must offer this training on initial assignment, then at least annually. In addition, laboratory and production facility personnel s must receive specialized initial training.

13. Maintain employee medical and training records.

    13.1. The employer also must maintain a Sharps Injury Log unless classified as an exempt industry under OSHA's standard on Recording and Reporting Occupational Injuries and Illnesses.

HOW CAN I GET MORE INFORMATION?

OSHA's website provides more in depth information on the Bloodborne Pathogens:

www.osha.gov/SLTC/bloodbornepathogens

U.S. DEPARTMENT OF LABOR

Occupational Safety and Health Administration 2002

This is one of a series of informational fact sheets highlighting OSHA programs, policies, or standards. It does not impose any new compliance requirements or carry the force of legal opinion. For compliance requirements of OSHA standards or regulations, refer to *Title 29 of the Code of Federal Regulations.*

This information must be made available to sensory-impaired individuals upon request. Voice phone: (202) 693-1999. See also OSHA's website at *www.osha.gov*

NUCLEAR MEDICINE
SECTION B5.   ADMINISTRATIVE AND OTHER PROTOCOLS
B5.9   Communicable Diseases

PROCEDURE:
This facility will not knowingly allow an employee who has a communicable disease that may pose a risk to patients and/or other personnel to continue their job responsibilities. If it is determined that an employee has a communicable disease:

1. The Medical Director, as it relates to his/her current responsibilities, will evaluate the employee's illness.
2. If appropriate, the employee will be relieved of their duties until illness no longer poses a risk to patients and other personnel.
3. If appropriate, and if reassignment options are available, the employee may be temporarily reassigned to other areas in the facility that does not pose a risk to patients and/or other employee.
4. Employees, who are ill, may be asked to pursue appropriate treatment with their personal physician.
5. Employees may be asked to provide a "return to work" statement from their personal physician when treatment is complete.
6. This faculty's Medical Director has the final decision making authority as to employee's ability to return to their original position.
7. To prevent the spread of communicable disease, employees shall demonstrate good personal hygiene and be free of communicable disease.
8. Employees with febrile respiratory or gastrointestinal illness should not have patient contact.
9. Any employee infected with varicella virus (chicken pox) should remain at home until all vesicles are dry and crusted, usually 5-6 days.
10. The employees' physician, if involved with direct patient care, should evaluate employees with shingles.
11. Any employee with herpetic whitlow (herpes simplex – hand) should avoid all patient contact or wear gloves until all vesicles are crusted.

NUCLEAR MEDICINE
SECTION B5.   ADMINISTRATIVE AND OTHER PROTOCOLS
B5.10   Hazardous Materials

PROCEDURE:
Completion of an MSDS (Material Safety Data Sheet) form is required for all hazardous materials.

1. Personnel must know when they are handling hazardous materials to ensure adequate protection and compliance with the proper safety procedures.
2. The Hazard Communication Standard created by OSHA requires that employers who use hazardous substances must make Material Safety Data Sheets (MSDS) available for employee use and reference, and provide appropriate warning labels on containers of hazardous substances within the facility.
3. An MSDS contains precautions for handling and using harmful substances and includes information such as health hazards, fire and explosion hazards, physical characteristics, hazardous ingredients, personal protective equipment, and spill procedures. *(See 29 CFR 1910.1450)*

The MSDS is usually prepared by the manufacturer or distributor of a hazardous substance.

The Hazard Communication Standard requires that the following categories of information be written in English on an MSDS form:

1. The Identity of the Substance:
    1.1.   Required information on the identity of the material as given on the product label.
    1.2.   Chemical and any common names
    1.3.   Mixtures to include chemical and common name(s) of the ingredients
    1.4.   Carcinogens to include those contents which comprise greater that 0.1%.

2. Physical and Chemical Characteristics:
    2.1.   the physical and chemical characteristics of the hazardous substance such as whether it is a liquid, gas, or solid,
    2.2.   and data pertaining to characteristics such as vapor pressure and flash point.
3. How the product will act under a variety of temperatures and conditions
4. If the material has an odor (and at what level the odor becomes noticeable)
5. The color of the material
6. Other items about the material's behavior

7. Physical Hazards to include:
    7.1.   Potential for fire, explosions, or reactions
    7.2.   Recommended extinguishing media (water, foam, dry chemical, carbon dioxide, graphite, etc).
8. Health Hazards to include:
    8.1.   Signs and symptoms of exposure (such as rash or burning of the eyes and throat)
    8.2.   Breathing difficulties that may occur
    8.3.   Routes of Entry: (potential routes of entry into the human body)
    8.4.   Absorption
    8.5.   Ingestion
    8.6.   Inhalation
    8.7.   Injection
    8.8.   Permissible Exposure Limits:
    8.9.   OSHA Permissible Exposure Limit [PEL]),
    8.10.   the American Conference of Governmental Industrial Hygienists (ACGIH) Threshold Limit Value (TLV),
    8.11.   and any other exposure limit recommended by the manufacturer, distributor, or employer preparing the MSDS must be given if such values are available.
    8.12.   Maximum exposure a worker should have to the substance during an eight-hour working day, as expressed in parts per million (ppm) in air.
    8.13.   TLV (recommended level) set by the ACGIH, which are advisory guidelines that are revised each year as more information becomes available for different chemicals.
9. Carcinogens:
    9.1.   Material listed in the National Toxicology Program (NTP) Annual Report on Carcinogens or that which has been found to be a potential carcinogen by OSHA or the International Agency for Research on Cancer).
10. Safe Handling:
    10.1.   Any generally applicable precautions for safe handling and use of the product that are known to the individual who prepares the MSDS.
    10.2.   Appropriate hygienic practices or protective measures during repair and maintenance of contaminated equipment.
    10.3.   Procedures for spills and leaks of the material.
    10.4.   First Aid Procedures to be used on a person who is exposed to the product.
    10.5.   Date of Preparation
    10.6.   Manufacturer Information:
    10.7.   Name, address and telephone number of the chemical
    10.8.   Manufacturer or responsible party who prepared the MSDS).

INSERT SAFETY DATA SHEETS
MSDS
MANUFACTURER
MATERIAL SAFETY DATA SHEETS
PRESCRIBING INFORMATION

NOTES

NUCLEAR MEDICINE
SECTION B5.   ADMINISTRATIVE AND OTHER PROTOCOLS
B5.11   Medical Emergencies

PROCEDURE:

GENERAL EMERGENCY CARE:

1. If a patient appears in distress while on the treadmill, push the emergency stop button
2. If there is time, gradually slow the belt down.
3. While still hooked up to the EKG monitor, have the patient lie down on the exam table and monitor the patient for rhythm changes.
4. If pharmacological infusion is in progress at the time of the distress, termination of the infusion may be necessary per the physician's discretion.
5. Push the red stop button on the pump.
6. If an event of fainting occurs, elevate the legs and use the ammonia inhalant taped to the EKG machine to attempt revival.
7. Keep the patient calm at all times.

PROCEDURES & RESUSCITATION EQUIPMENT:

1. A cardiologist must be present in the facility at all times when exercise testing is conducted.
2. A cardiologist is to be called if any of the following situations are present:
    2.1. Ongoing chest pain
    2.2. Respiratory distress
    2.3. Syncope or pre-syncope
    2.4. Significant arrhythmia
    2.5. Active ECG changes
    2.6. Sever hypotension or hypertension
3. The ACLS-NP, RN, or physician in charge will direct resuscitation efforts according to ACLS guidelines as adjusted by appropriate clinical judgment.
4. In the case of cardiac arrest or major clinical emergency, the following guidelines will be observed:
    4.1. Cardiologist is to be called immediately
    4.2. Supervising physician, NP, or RN must follow Advanced Cardiac Life Support guidelines.
    4.3. Staff is to dial 911 for EMS to be deployed.
    4.4. All available staff members are to assist as directed

     4.5.   Staff member will go outside and direct EMS squad to appropriate location.

     4.6.   When patient stability is achieved events are to be documented in patient record

5. All staff supervising exercise testing will have current Advanced Cardiac Life Support (ACLS) certification.
6. All clinical staff (Nuclear Technologists, ECG technicians) will have current basic life support (BLS).
7. A crash cart and defibrillator must be available in the room where exercise testing is conducted.
8. Emergency drug cart, oxygen, and equipment must be current and in good working order at all times.
9. The defibrillator function is to be checked daily prior to start of any testing
10. A preventative maintenance check must be conducted on the defibrillator on a semi-annual basis
11. The crash cart must be evaluated for expiration of drugs and presence of required emergency drugs at the end of each month or after each crash cart usage.

PROCEDURE FOR CPR OR EMERGENT CARE

1. First personnel to recognize Code Assist Situation will activate emergency response system and then begin CPR if necessary.
2. All available RN's or other BLS certified staff will respond to all Code Assists.
3. Second personnel will respond and if necessary call 911, contact physician and assist, if needed, in CPR.
4. Available personnel will take Code Notes

     4.1.   RN or Nuclear Technologist if possible and assist, as needed,

5. Prepare patient for transport to hospital.
6. Specific Instructions for Squad:

     6.1.   Verify location and specify entrance

     6.2.   Designate a staff person to meet the squad at the entrance to direct them to the emergency location.

Code Plan of Action

B5.11   CODE PLAN OF ACTION SIGN

RECEPTIONIST

GET DOCTOR ! ! !

GO INTO EXAM ROOM AND GET THE NEAREST DOCTOR

Dial 911

- CLEAR ALL HALLWAYS
  - *Keep Access To Stress Room Clear For Emergency Personnel*
- WAIT BY ENTRANCE TO DIRECT EMERGENCY PERSONNEL TO AREA
- DIRECT SQUARD TO STRESS ROOM

NURSE/BCS/ACLS PERSONNEL

- REPORT IMMEDIATELY TO EMERGENCY AREA
- INITIATE ACLS
- MONITOR EKG
- PUSH IV DRUGS
- RUN CODE UNTIL DOCTOR ARRIVES
- REMAIN IN ROOM WHILE CODE IS ONGOING
- EXCEPT TO KEEP FAMILY INFORMED AS NEEDED

NUCLEAR MEDICINE TECHNOLOGIST

- REPORT IMMEDIATELY TO EMERGENCY AREA
- INITIATE ACLS
- START OXYGEN
- PLACE 02 ON PATIENT
- START IV FLUID
- START 2ND LINE
- TAKE VITALS

ALL OTHER PERSONNEL

- GET NURSE
- INITIATE ACLS
  - CHART ON CODE SHEET
  - ASSIST WITH BLOOD PRESSURE

NOTES

NUCLEAR MEDICINE
SECTION B5. ADMINISTRATIVE AND OTHER PROTOCOLS
B5.12   Patients with special needs

PROCEDURE:
1. All staff is competent in the care of patients with vision impairments.
2. All staff is trained for handling special medical needs such as IV's, wounds, catheters, and Oxygen tanks and tubing.
3. Patients confined to a wheelchair or cart will be lifted using a draw-sheet technique.
4. If a patient becomes violent, threatening, or combative, the supervising physician must be notified, as will the facility security department if necessary.

The hearing impaired will be provided with a person proficient in sign language for their visit to the department.

Translator Contact_____

Address: _____

City: _____ State: _____ Zip:_____

Home Phone: _____ Work Phone: _____ Cell Phone: _____

Web Site: _____E-mail: _____

Patient in need of foreign language translator.

Translator Contact_____

Address: _____

City: _____ State: _____ Zip:_____

Home Phone: _____ Work Phone: _____ Cell Phone: _____

Web Site: _____E-mail: _____

NOTES

NUCLEAR MEDICINE
SECTION B5.   ADMINISTRATIVE AND OTHER PROTOCOLS
B5.13   Non-radioactive Drug Use
Non-Radioactive Pharmaceuticals

PROCEDURE:
PREPARATION
1. All pharmaceuticals must be prepared according to package insert and under the Medical Director's supervision.
2. Storage
3. All pharmaceuticals must be stored in a locked cabinet or crash cart.
4. Only authorized (per the Medical Director) personnel will have access to locked areas storing pharmaceuticals.

ADMINISTRATION
1. All patient doses must be determined using standard protocols or by written directive from the physician.
2. The health care provider is responsible for prescribing the pharmaceutical and must clearly identify each patient dose via prescription or protocol.
3. The patient must be properly identified according to the Patient Identification protocol.
4. The identity, dosage, expiration date/time, and route must be verified prior to administration.
5. There must be clear documentation of the substance, amount, route, site, time and the identity of the person administering.

INVESTIGATIONAL DRUGS AT PRESENT,
    ☐ There are investigational drugs being used at this facility
    ☐ There are no investigational drugs being used at this facility

NUCLEAR MEDICINE
> **SECTION B5.   ADMINISTRATIVE AND OTHER PROTOCOLS**
> B5.14   Adverse Drug Events (Medical Events)

PROCEDURE:
RADIOPHARMACEUTICALS AND OTHER MEDICATIONS
While the risk of an adverse drug event is minimal as to radiopharmaceuticals used in this facility for diagnostic cardiac imaging, the following procedure is recognized:
1. Any adverse reaction to a radiopharmaceutical injection or any other medication must be assessed by the supervising physician.
2. A thorough medical exam of the patient involved may be performed immediately following the incident with emergency action taken, if applicable.
   > 2.1.1. The supervising physician will document all treatment on the
3. Incident Form and sign/date the document.
   3.1.   *See B5.15 Drug Administration Errors, ,Incident/Occurrence Forms*
   3.2.   This document must also be reviewed by the Medical Director.
   3.3.   Copies will be kept on file in the Nuclear Medicine Department.

MEDICAL EVENTS
Adverse Drug Reactions is defined as "Medical Event"

DOCUMENTATION OF MEDICATION ERRORS
AND ADVERSE DRUG REACTIONS

1. Medication errors and Adverse Drug Reaction (ADR) are to be reported consistent with:
   > ∴ *B5.15Drug Administration Errors*
   > ∴ *Incident/Occurrence Policy*
   > ∴ *Incident/Occurrence Forms*
   > B5.15   Incident Occurrence Report
2. It is essential that staff assist in the collection of information regarding medication errors and Adverse Drug Reactions. Errors provide opportunities to identify system problems that contribute to errors and Adverse Drug Reactions. and improve practices that will reduce errors and Adverse Drug Reactions..
3. A medication error is defined as medication administration that deviates from the original physician's order or standard clinic policy and procedure.
4. An adverse drug reaction is defined as any response to a drug which is noxious and unintended and that occurs at doses used in man for prophylaxis, diagnosis, and therapy.
5. A reportable Adverse Drug Reactions is any suspected Adverse Drug Reactions. which causes a change in drug therapy (including corrective measures such as antidotes), causes discontinuation of drug therapy?

PROCEDURE STATEMENTS
1. At finding of a Medication Error or Adverse Drug Reactions, the Technologist, RN, LPN, Staff should contact the physician and must complete

B5.15 Drug Administration Errors
- Incident/Occurrence Policy
- Incident/Occurrence Forms
- B5.15   Incident Occurrence Report

2. The completed Unusual Occurrence Report should be given to the appropriate authority by the end of the shift during the incident occurred or was discovered.
3. The appropriate manager reviews the incident report and completes follow-up.
4. The completed Occurrence Report should be directed to the Medical Director.

CATEGORIES OF MEDICATION ADMINISTRATION ERRORS:
1. Omission: Failure to administer an ordered dose.
   1.1.   No error has occurred if the patient refuses to take the medication or if the dose is not administered because of contraindications
   1.2.   Physician must be notified and incident documented in medical record.
2. Incorrect patient.
3. Incorrect drug administered.
4. Duplication/Extra dose of medication given.
5. Incorrect IV solution.
6. Incorrect dose.
7. Incorrect time
   7.1.   medication is not administered within the established period.
8. Incorrect rate.
9. Incorrect route
   9.1.   Included is dose given via the correct route but at the wrong site
   9.2.   e.g. left eye vs. right eye).
10. Incorrect preparation
    10.1.   incorrect preparation of the medication dose.
    10.2.   e.g. incorrect dilution or reconstitution
    10.3.   not shaking suspension
    10.4.   issuing expired drug
    10.5.   exposure of light-sensitive drug to light
    10.6.   mixing drugs that are visually or chemically incompatible
11. Incorrect dosage form
    11.1.   Administration of a drug by the correct route but in a different dosage form than specified by the physician.
    11.2.   e.g. use of an ophthalmic ointment when a solution was ordered.

12. It is generally not an error to purposefully alter
    12.1.   e.g. crushing of a tablet
    12.2.   or substitute e.g. liquid for a tablet oral dosage to facilitate administration.
13. No error.

SERIOUS ADVERSE EVENT REPORTING

A *serious adverse event* (SAE) is a medical condition that results in death, is life threatening requires inpatient hospitalization or prolongs an existing hospitalization, creates persistent or significant disability or incapacity, or results in a congenital anomaly or birth defect.

ADVERSE DRUG REACTIONS CLASSIFICATIONS

Level		
0	Report does not constitute ADR	Should not report
1	Causes no harm to patient/ no change in treatment	Report
2	Result in need for increased monitoring Suspected drug was held, discontinued, or otherwise changed	Report
3	Resulted in a change in vital sign or need for additional lab work	Report
4	Result in need for treatment, increased length of stay, or reason for admission	Report
5	Result in need for intensive medical care (monitored bed, ICU, intubation) or permanent patient harm	Report
6	Contributed to the death of the patient	Report

NUCLEAR MEDICINE POLICY & PROCEDURES

NUCLEAR MEDICINE
B5.14   Adverse Reaction Table
ADVERSE EFFECTS OF RADIOPHARMACEUTICALS AND OTHER MEDICATIONS

RADIOPHARMACEUTICAL	TRADE NAME	SIDE EFFECTS, COMMENTS & OTHER REACTIONS
57Co-cyanocobalamin	Rubratope-57, Dicopac kit	None.
51Cr-sodium chromate	Chromitope	Erythema, flushing, hypertension, tachycardia and diaphoresis.
18F-fludeoxyglucose,FDG, fluorodeoxyglucose		None.
59Fe-ferrous citrate		None.
67Ga-gallium citrate	Neoscan	Nausea, vomiting, erythema, flushing, diffuse rash, pruritus, hives/urticaria, respiratory reaction, tachycardia, syncope, fainting, dizziness, vertigo, facial swelling, metallic taste, dyspnea, salty taste.
111In-capromab pendetide	ProstaScint	Increase in bilirubin, hypotension, hypertension, injection site reactions, elevated liver enzymes (could be due to tumor), pruritus, fever, rash, headache, myalgia, asthenia, burning sensation in thigh, shortness of breath, alterations of taste, production of hama by the recipient.
111In-indium oxyquinoline, Oxine		Fever, diffuse rash, pruritus and hives/urticaria.
111In-pentetate DTPA	MPI-DTPA	Fever, nausea, vomiting, erythema, flushing, pruritus, hives/urticaria, cardiac arrest, hypertension, headache, aseptic meningitis; one death 20 min postinjection.
111In-pentetreotide	Octreoscan	Fever, nausea, erythema, flushing, hypotension, bradycardia, dizziness, vertigo, headache, diaphoresis, arthralgia and asthenia, one case of anemia.
111In-satumomab pendetide	OncoScint CR/OV	Chills, fever, nausea, erythema, flushing, diffuse rash, pruritus, chest pain, tightness or heaviness, hypertension, hypotension, dizziness, vertigo, headache, diaphoresis, arthralgia and asthenia, confusion, diarrhea, hypothermia, bradycardia, vasodilatation,angioedema, production of hama by the recipient.
123I-iobenguane metaiodobenzylguanidine, MIBG		Nausea, erythema, flushing, hypertension, respiratory reaction, syncope or faintness, dizziness and vertigo, tachypnea.
123I-iodohippurate sodium	Nephroflow, Nephropure	Nausea, vomiting, diffuse rash, pruritus, hives/urticaria and hypotension.
123I-sodium iodide		Nausea, vomiting, diffuse rash, pruritus, hives/urticaria, chest pain, tightness or heaviness, respiratory reaction, tachycardia, syncope or faintness and headache, tachypnea; parosmia.
125I-iodinated albumin (IHSA, iodinated human serum albumin)		Diffuse rash.

RADIOPHARMACEUTICAL	TRADE NAME	SIDE EFFECTS, COMMENTS & OTHER REACTIONS
125I-sodium iothalamate	Glofil	None.
131I-iobenguane metaiodobenzylguanidine, MIBG		Erythema, flushing, diaphoresis and metallic taste, tingling of arms and face.
131I-iodinated albumin	RISA, Radioinated serum, albumin, Megatope	None.
131I-iodohippurate sodium	Hipputope, Hippuran	Nausea, vomiting, pruritus hives/urticaria, hypertension, respiratory reaction, tachycardia, syncope/fainting, diaphoresis, anaphylaxis, facial swelling, dyspnea; "cold sweat", pallor; amaurosis fugax.
131I-sodium iodide	Iodotope	Chills, nausea, vomiting, pruritus, hives/urticaria, chest pain, tightness or heaviness, tachycardia, headache, dizziness.
131I-6-beta iodomethyl-18-norcholesterol	NP-59	Nausea, vomiting, erythema, flushing, chest pain, tightness or heaviness, hypertension, respiratory reaction, tachycardia, dizziness, headaches, diaphoresis, facial swelling, abdominal pain, metallic taste, frozen tongue, dyspnea.
81mKr-krypton		None.
13N-ammonia		None.
32P-chromic phosphate suspension	Phosphocol	Chills, fever, nausea, vomiting, chest pain, tightness or heaviness, respiratory reaction, abdominal pain, dyspnea, sore throat, cough, pleuritis, myelosuppression.
32P-sodium phosphate		Myelosuppression, bone pain from the flare phenomenon.
82Rb-rubidium		None.
153Sm-lexidronam	Quadramet	Myelosuppression, bone pain from the flare phenomenon.
89Sr-strontium chloride	Metastron	Chills, fever, myelosuppression, bone pain from the flare phenomenon.
99mTc-albumin colloid	Microlite	Chills, nausea, erythema, flushing, diffuse rash, pruritus, hypertension, hypotension, respiratory reaction, tachycardia, dizziness, vertigo, diaphoresis, anaphylaxis, abdominal pain, myelosuppression (injectate also included mdp and soluble albumin for cases with anaphylaxis).
99mTc-albumin (HSA, human serum, albumin)		Chills, fever, erythema, flushing, diffuse rash, hypotension, tachycardia, dizziness, vertigo, facial swelling, tachypnea, malaise, dyspnea.
99mTc-arcitumomab	CEA-Scan	Transient eosinophilia, nausea, bursitis, urticaria, pruritus, headache, nausea, fever, one grand mal seizure, hama production by the recipient.

RADIOPHARMACEUTICAL	TRADE NAME	SIDE EFFECTS, COMMENTS & OTHER REACTIONS
99mTc-bicisate dihydrochloride (ethyl cysteinate dimer, ECD)	Neurolite	Nausea, diffuse rash, chest pain, tightness or heaviness, respiratory reaction, seizures, syncope or faintness, dizziness, vertigo, headache, cyanosis and asthenia, neurologic adverse events may have been related to underlying disease, including hallucinations, parosmia, also cardiac failure; respiratory arrest.
99mTc-disofenin	Hepatolite	None.
99mTc-exametazime (hexamethylpropylene amine oxine, HMPAO)	Ceretec	Fever, erythema, flushing, diffuse rash, hypertension, hypotension, respiratory reaction, seizures, diaphoresis, cyanosis, anaphylaxis, facial swelling, abdominal pain, dyspnea with myoclonus (labeled wbc).
99mTc-gluceptate	Glucoscan, Technescan, Gluceptate	Chills, nausea, erythema, flushing, diffuse rash, hives/urticaria, respiratory reaction, tachycardia, seizures, dizziness, vertigo, headache, diaphoresis.
99mTc-lidofenin	Technescan HIDA	Chills, nausea.
99mTc-macroaggregated albumin (MAA)	AN-MAA, Macrotec, MPI-MAA, Pulmolite, Technescan MAA	Chills, nausea, erythema, flushing, diffuse rash, pruritus, hives/urticaria, cardiac arrest, chest pain, tightness or heaviness, hypertension, hypotension, respiratory reaction, tachycardia, syncope or faintness, diaphoresis, cyanosis, anaphylaxis, metallic taste, dyspnea; throat tightness; arm numbness; parosmia.
99mTc-mebrofenin	Choletec	Hives/urticaria.
99mTc-medronate (MDP, methylene diphosphonate)	Osteolite, Technescan, MDP, AN-MDP, MPI-MDP	Chills, fever, nausea, vomiting, erythema, flushing, diffuse rash, pruritus, hives, urticaria, cardiac arrest, chest pain, tightness or heaviness, hypertension, hypotension, respiratory reaction, tachycardia, seizures, syncope or fainting, dizziness, vertigo, headache, diaphoresis, anaphylaxis, abdominal pain, metallic taste, asthenia, pain/burning at Site, photophobia, one death secondary to cardiac arrhythmia.
99mTc-mertiatide (MAG3, mercaptoacetyl-glyclyglyclyglycine)	Technescan MAG3	Nausea, vomiting, erythema, flushing, syncope or faintness, sore, thick throat.
99mTc-oxidronate (HDP, hydroxymethylene diphosphonate)	Osteoscan-HDP	Nausea, vomiting, erythema, flushing, diffuse rash, pruritus, chest pain, tightness or heaviness, heartburn, seizures, diaphoresis, facial swelling.

RADIOPHARMACEUTICAL	TRADE NAME	SIDE EFFECTS, COMMENTS & OTHER REACTIONS
99mTc-pentetate (DTPA, diethylenetriaminepentaacetic acid)	Technescan DTPA, AN DTPA, MPI-DTPA, Techniplex	Chills, nausea, erythema, flushing, diffuse rash, pruritus, hives/urticaria, hypertension, hypotension, respiratory reaction, tachycardia, syncope or faintness, headache, cyanosis, anaphylaxis, arthralgia, pain, burning at inj. Site, cough; wheezing; trisodium salt can cause neurologic signs if given inthrathecally.
99mTc-pyrophosphate (PYP) and Sodium Pyrophosphate)	Pyrolite, Technescan PYP, Phosphotec, MPI, Pyrophosphate, AN Pyrotec, Ultratag	Chills, fever, nausea, vomiting, erythema, flushing, diffuse rash, pruritus, hives/urticaria, chest pain, tightness or heaviness, hypotension, respiratory reaction, syncope or faintness, dizziness, vertigo, pain/burning at inj. Site, tinnitus.
99mTc-sestamibi	Cardiolite, Mirluma	Nausea, erythema, flushing, diffuse rash, pruritus, seizures, headache, metallic taste, tingling.
99mTc-sodium pertechnetate	Minitec, UltratecKow	Chills, nausea, vomiting, diffuse rash, pruritus, hives/urticaria, chest pain, tightness or heaviness, hypertension, dizziness, vertigo, headache, diaphoresis, anaphylaxis.
99mTc-succimer (DMSA, dimercaptosuccinic acid)	MPI-DMSA, Nephroscint	Nausea erythema, flushing, syncope or faintness, abdominal pain.
99mTc-sulfur colloid	AN-Sulfur Colloid, TechneColl, TcSC, Tesuloid	Chills, fever, nausea, vomiting, erythema, flushing, diffuse rash, pruritus, hives/urticaria, cardiac arrest, chest pain, tightness or heaviness, hypertension, hypotension, respiratory reaction, tachycardia, bradycardia, seizures, syncope or faintness, dizziness, vertigo, headache, diaphoresis, cyanosis, anaphylaxis, arthralgia, pain/burning at inj. Site, wheezing, dyspnea, choking; sneezing, itchy throat, parasthesia, weakness.
99mTc-tetrofosmin	Myoview	Angina, hypertension, torsades de pointes (these three probably occurred because of underlying heart disease); vomiting, abdominal discomfort, cutaneous allergy, hypotension, dyspnea, metallic taste, burning of mouth, unusual odor, mild leukocytosis.
201Tl-thallous chloride		Fever, erythema, flushing, diffuse rash, pruritus, hypotension.
127Xe-xenon		None.
133Xe-xenon		None.

NUCLEAR MEDICINE

>**SECTION B5.** **ADMINISTRATIVE AND OTHER PROTOCOLS**
>B5.15 Drug Administration Errors
>Incident/Occurrence Policy
>Incident/Occurrence Report
>Misadministration and Recordable Events

PROCEDURE:

Misadministration of a diagnostic radiopharmaceutical is defined as a *"Medical Event"* Including:

1. A dose that differs from the prescribed dose, or the dose that would have resulted from the prescribed dosage, by more than 0.05 Sv (5 rem) effective dose equivalent, (0.5 Sv (50 rem) to an organ or tissue), or 0.5 Sv (50 rem) shallow dose equivalent to the skin, where:
    1.1. the total dose delivered differs from the prescribed dose by 20 percent or more;
    1.2. individual organ to:
    1.3. the wrong patient
    1.4. the wrong radiopharmaceutical
    1.5. the wrong route of administration
    1.6. an administered dosage that differs significantly from the prescribed dosage.

2. Records of Misadministration must be kept for 10 years and include:
    2.1. Names of Individuals involved in the Medical Event
    2.2. Social security or identification number of the patient
    2.3. Copy of the report of misadministration filed with the state
    2.4. Details of effect on patient
    2.5. Action taken, if any, to prevent reoccurrence
    2.6. Referring physician and patient must be notified within 24 hours after the misadministration.
    2.7. If referring physician cannot be notified within 24 hours, patient notification may also be delayed.
    2.8. There must be no delay on appropriate medical care due to delay of notification.
    2.9. If patient is notified, patient must be provided a written report of the incident within 15 days including consequences that may affect the patient.

NOTIFICATIONS, REPORTS, AND RECORDS OF MEDICAL EVENTS

A registrant shall report any medical event, except for an event that results from patient intervention, in which the administration of radiation results in one or more of the events or involves the wrong patient, wrong treatment site, or wrong mode of treatment.

A licensee shall report any medical event, except for an event that results from patient intervention, in which the administration of radioactive material or radiation from radioactive material results in:

1. A dose that differs from the prescribed dose, or the dose that would have resulted from the prescribed dosage, by more than 0.05 Sv (5 rem) effective dose equivalent, (0.5 Sv (50 rem) to an organ or tissue), or 0.5 Sv (50 rem) shallow dose equivalent to the skin, where:

    1.1. the total dose delivered differs from the prescribed dose by 20 percent or more;

    1.2. the total dosage delivered differs from the prescribed dosage by 20 percent or more or falls outside the prescribed dosage range; or

    1.3. the fractionated dose delivered differs from the prescribed dose, for a single fraction, by 50 percent or more;

2. A dose that exceeds 0.05 Sv (5 rem) effective dose equivalent, 0.5 Sv (50 rem) to an organ or tissue, or 0.5 Sv (50 rem) shallow dose equivalent to the skin from any of the following:

    2.1. an administration of a wrong radioactive drug;

    2.2. an administration of a radioactive drug by the wrong route of administration;

    2.3. an administration of a dose or dosage to the wrong individual or human research subject;

    2.4. an administration of a dose or dosage delivered by the wrong mode of treatment; or

    2.5. a leaking sealed source; or

    2.6. a dose to the skin or an organ or tissue other than the treatment site that exceeds 0.5 Sv (50 rem) to an organ or tissue and 50 percent or more of the dose expected from the administration defined in the written directive (excluding, for permanent implants, seeds that were implanted in the correct site but migrated outside the treatment site).

A licensee shall report any event resulting from intervention of a patient or human research subject in which the administration of radioactive material results or will result in unintended permanent functional damage to an organ or a physiological system, as determined by a physician.

1. The written report shall include
    1.1.   the licensee's name;
    1.2.   the prescribing physician's name;
    1.3.   a brief description of the event;
    1.4.   why the event occurred;
    1.5.   the effect on the individual who received the administration;
    1.6.   what improvements are needed to prevent recurrence; actions taken to prevent recurrence;
    1.7.   whether the licensee notified the individual, or the individual's responsible relative or guardian, and if not, why not,
    1.8.   and if the individual was notified, what information was provided to the individual.

2. The report shall not include the individual's name or other information that could lead to identification of the individual.
    To meet the requirements of this Section, the notification of the medical event may be made to the individual or instead to that individual's responsible relative or guardian, when appropriate.

3. The licensee shall notify the referring physician and also notify the individual who is the subject of the medical event no later than 24 hours after its discovery, unless the referring physician personally informs the licensee either that he will inform the individual or that, based on medical judgment, telling the individual would be harmful.

4. The licensee is not required to notify the individual without first consulting the referring physician. If the referring physician or the affected individual cannot be reached within 24 hours, the licensee shall notify the individual as soon as possible thereafter.

5. The licensee may not delay any appropriate medical care for the individual, including any necessary remedial care as a result of the medical event, because of any delay in notification.
    5.1.   To meet the requirements of this Paragraph, the notification to the individual who is the subject of the medical event may be made instead to that individual's responsible relative or guardian. If a verbal notification is made, the licensee shall inform the individual, or appropriate responsible relative or guardian, that a written description of the event can be obtained from the licensee upon request.

6. The licensee shall provide such a written description if requested.

7. If the individual was notified, the licensee shall also furnish, within 15 days after discovery of the medical event, written report to the individual by sending either:
    7.1.   a copy of the report that was submitted to the department; or
    7.2.   a brief description of both the event and the consequences as they may affect the individual, provided a statement is included that the report submitted to the department can be obtained from the licensee.

8. Each licensee shall retain a record of each medical event for five years. The record shall contain
    8.1.   the names of all individuals involved
    8.2.   including the prescribing physician, allied health personnel, the individual affected by the medical event, and the individual's referring physician
    8.3.   the individual's driver's license or state identification number and the issuing state,
    8.4.   a brief description of the medical event, why it occurred, the effect on the individual,
    8.5.   what improvements are needed to prevent recurrence, and the actions taken to prevent recurrence.

Aside from the notification requirement, nothing in this Section affects any rights or duties of licensees and physicians in relation to each other, the individual, or the individual's responsible relatives or guardians.

A LICENSEE SHALL:

1. Annotate a copy of the report provided to the department with:

      1.1.   the name of the individual who is the subject of the event; and

      1.2.   the social security number or other identification number, if one has been assigned, of the individual who is the subject of the event; and

      1.3.   provide a copy of the annotated report to the referring physician, if other than the licensee, no later than 15 days after the discovery of the event.

CRITERIA FOR RECORDABLE EVENT OR A MISADMINISTRATION

PROCEDURE	RECORDABLE EVENT	MISADMINISTRATION
All diagnostic radiopharmaceuticals (including <30 µCi NaI, I-125 or I-131)	None	Wrong patient Radiopharmaceutical route, or dosage and Dose >5 rem Effective Dose Equivalent or 50 rem to organ
Sodium Iodide Radiopharmaceuticals (where >30 µCi NaI, I-125 or I-131)	Admin dosage differs by >10% prescribed dosage and >15 µCi Without written directive Without daily dosage record	Wrong patient Wrong pharmaceutical Admin dosage differs by >20% prescribed dosage and >30 µCi
Therapeutic Radiopharmaceuticals	Admin dosage differs by >10% prescribed dosage and >15 µCi Without written directive Without daily dosage record	Wrong patient Wrong pharmaceutical Admin dosage differs by >20% prescribed dosage and >30 µCi

NOTES

NUCLEAR MEDICINE

SECTION B5.   ADMINISTRATIVE AND OTHER PROTOCOLS
B5.15   Drug Administration Errors
                Incident/Occurrence Report
                Non-Radioactive Drug Administration Errors

PROCEDURE:

1. Immediately following the incident, the patient who is subject of the administration error will undergo appropriate emergency action and a thorough medical exam.

2. All drug administration errors must be followed by the completion of an
    Incident Occurrence Report
    prepared in a timely manner by the staff that made the administration error.

3. The *Incident Occurrence Report* will be reviewed and signed by the Technical Director and the staff involved.

4. The supervising physician will document all treatment on the *Incident Occurrence Report* with signature and date.

5. The *Incident Occurrence Report* must be reviewed by the Medical Director and copy entered in file in the Nuclear Department.

    5.1.   Names of all staff involved in the occurrence.

    5.2.   Social security or identification number of the patient, visitor, or employee.

    5.3.   Complete description of the occurrence to include date and time.

    5.4.   Any injury incurred by the involved person including documentation of physician evaluation

    5.5.   Name and signature of evaluating physician and/or Medical Director.

    5.6.   Names of all witnesses

6. The completed *Incident Occurrence Report* will be evaluated by the Medical Director for any necessary action.

7. A copy of the Occurrence Report form shall be kept on file with practice management for five (5) years.

NOTES

NUCLEAR MEDICINE
B5.1.5   INCIDENT OCCURRENCE REPORT

DATE OF REPORT:	
DATE OF OCURRENCE:	
NAMES OF ALL INVOLVED:	
EMPLOYEE:	
PATIENT:	
VISITOR :	
PERSON COMPLETING FORM:	
WITNESSESS:	
WITNESSESS:	

DESCRIPTION OF OCCURRENCE:

EVALUATING PHYSICIAN:	
PHYSICIAN OBSERVATIONS:	

RECCOMMENDED FOLLOWUP:

SIGNATURES:		DATE:
PHYSICIAN		
PERSON COMPLETING FORM:		
CLINICAL MANAGER		

NOTES

NUCLEAR MEDICINE
SECTION B6.   IMAGE INTERPRETATION AND REPORTING
B6.1   Report Generation Requirements

PROCEDURE:
Document the appropriateness, necessity, and performance of the procedure

ESSENTIALS OF REPORTS:
1. Study Identification
2. Patient name.
3. Other information to uniquely identify the patient, such as sex, date of birth, social security number, medical record number, or universal patient code.
4. Requesting physician and other appropriate health care providers such as the primary care physician.
5. Date of study.
6. Type of study
7. Study accession number (in a well integrated information system, the study
8. Accession number may not need to be visible).
9. History
10. Time of study, if relevant.
11. Completion dates and times.
12. Indications
13. Other relevant histories—see specific procedure guideline for details.
14. Information needed for billing such as referral number, patient status (e.g., inpatient/outpatient), or diagnostic codes (e.g. ICD-9-CM code)

PROCEDURE
Significant discrepancies between an initial and final report should be promptly reconciled by direct communication.
1. Radiopharmaceutical.
2. Administered dose.
3. Route of administration.
4. Timing of imaging relative to radiopharmaceutical administration.
5. Other drugs used, including name, dose, route, rate of administration, and timing relative to images.
6. Catheters or devices used.
7. Imaging technique, including alteration in normal procedure.
8. Complications or patient reactions.

DESCRIPTION OF FINDINGS
1. Significant positive findings as well as pertinent negative findings should be mentioned.
2. Image quality or other causes of study limitations (e.g., patient motion).
3. A reference range may be useful for quantitative values.
4. See individual guidelines for specifics.

IMPRESSION

1. A separate impression should be included for all but the shortest reports.
2. The impression should address the clinical indication for the scan.
3. Diagnoses, differential diagnoses, and judgments about the significance of the pertinent findings may be included in the impression.

COMMENTS

1. Study limitations.
2. Recommendations for further procedures, if appropriate.
3. Documentation of direct communication of results including the name of the physician or physician designate and time/date of contact.
4. Comments may be included in the Impression section, especially when brief.

ISSUES REQUIRING FURTHER CLARIFICATION

1. Findings
2. List the diagnosis to the highest level of specificity known at the time of billing
3. or, if no diagnosis is known, the pertinent symptom or sign that led to the procedure.
4. Results of examinations with critical results must be communicated to the referring physician as quickly as clinically indicated.
5. A record of the communication should be maintained.

GENERAL REQUIREMENTS

1. Exams must be interpreted with the final report provided by the Medical Director or a member of the medical staff
2. Interpretation must occur promptly after the study is completed as appropriate for the risk of clinically significant results.
3. Final reports must be signed manually or password protected electronically by the responsible physician.
4. All records are to be maintained confidentially for at least 3 years. *(or conform to State and Federal Laws)*
5. Final reports must be typed or computer generated.

FINAL REPORTS MUST ACCURATELY REFLECT THE CONTENT AND RESULTS OF THE STUDY

1. Type of study
2. History
3. Indication
4. Procedure
5. Findings
6. Impression
7. Completion dates and times.
8. Clinical information and indication for the study

9. Radionuclide images
10. Radioactive dose information
11. Stress or pharmacologic date to include EKG findings, symptoms and hemodynamic response (BP and HR)
12. Other imaging modality data for comparison if applicable
13. Previous exam data for comparison when applicable
14. Overview of positive or negative findings to include localization and quantification of abnormal image and stress findings
15. Reasons for limited exam
16. Overall succinct impression
17. Any need for additional studies based on finding
18. Identification and signature of interpreting physician

NOTES

NUCLEAR MEDICINE
B6.1.2   Interpretive Report Timeliness Requirements
Standards of Image Interpretation and Reporting

PROCEDURE:
Patient study report dissemination
Completed interpretation within 1 business day
Final report transmittal within 2 business days

ESSENTIALS OF REPORTS:
1. Title
2. Type of study
3. History
4. Indications
5. Procedure
6. Findings
7. Impression

∴ **Results of examinations with critical results must be communicated to the referring physician as quickly as clinically indicated.**
∴ **A record of the communication should be maintained.**

GENERAL REQUIREMENTS
1. Exams must be interpreted with the final report provided by the Medical Director or a member of the medical staff
2. Interpretation must occur promptly after the study is completed as appropriate for the risk of clinically significant results.
3. Final reports must be signed manually or password protected electronically by the responsible physician.
4. All records are to be maintained confidentially for at least 3 years.
5. Final reports must be typed or computer generated.
6. Final reports must accurately reflect the content and results of the study.

CONTENTS OF A NUCLEAR MEDICINE REPORT
1. Study identification
2. Patient name.
3. Other information to uniquely identify the patient, such as sex, date of birth, Social Security number, medical record number, or universal patient code.
4. Signed request by physician and other appropriate health care providers such as the primary care physician.
5. Date of study.
6. Time of study.
7. Study accession number (in a well-integrated information system, the study accession number may not need to be visible).
8. Completion dates and times.

9. Clinical information and indication for the study
10. Radionuclide images
11. Radioactive dose information
12. Stress or pharmacologic date to include EKG findings, symptoms and hemodynamic response (BP and HR)
13. Other imaging modality data for comparison if applicable
14. Previous exam data for comparison when applicable
15. Overview of positive or negative findings to include localization and quantification of abnormal image and stress findings
16. Reasons for limited exam
17. Overall succinct impression
18. Any need for additional studies based on finding
19. Identification and signature of interpreting physician

PATIENT STUDY REPORT DISSEMINATION

∴ *Completed interpretation within 1 business day*
∴ *Final report transmittal within 2 business days*

PATIENT STUDY REPORT DISSEMINATION

∴ *Completed interpretation within 1 business day*
∴ *Final report transmittal within 2 business days*

1. Record of date and time of studies and final reports were generated and signed manually or electronically (with password protection) by the interpreting physician to be called *Final Report Log.*
2. *Final Report Log* will be reviewed quarterly by Medical Director or his designee to ensure that, final reports are generated within two working days.
3. Medical Director will address deficiencies during quarterly quality assessment meetings.
   B6.1.3 An interpretation (initial or final) must be available within two (2) working days of the examination. An initial interpretation may be in the form of paper, digital storage or accessible voice system.

   B6.1.4 The final report must be reviewed and signed manually or electronically (with password protection) by the interpreting physician (who must be the medical director or a qualified member of the medical staff).
   - *Stamped signatures or signing by non-physician staff is unacceptable. In unusual circumstances, when the interpreting physician is not available, another qualified member of the medical staff may sign for them, if they choose to take such responsibility.*

   B6.1.5 The final signed report must be transmitted to the referring health care provider within 4 working days.

Accepted by: _____ (Initials) Date_____

NUCLEAR MEDICINE

B6.1.2   Interpretive Report Timeliness Quality Assurance
Maintain Timely Image Interpretation and Reporting

PROCEDURE:

To comply with ICANL diagnostic procedure interpreting guidelines, facility will generate a quarterly record of date and time of studies and date final reports were generated and signed manually or electronically (with password protection) by the interpreting physician to be called *Final Report Log.* *(Log may be reviewed on computer monthly or quarterly)*

PATIENT STUDY REPORT DISSEMINATION
Completed interpretation within 1 business day
Final report transmittal within 2 business days

Final Report Log will be reviewed quarterly by Medical Director or as his designee to ensure that final reports are generated within two working days.
Medical Director will address deficiencies during quarterly quality assessment meetings.

> *B6.1.3 An interpretation (initial or final) must be available within two (2) working days of the examination. An initial interpretation may be in the form of paper, digital storage or accessible voice system.*

> *B6.1.4 The final report must be reviewed and signed manually or electronically (with password protection) by the interpreting physician (who must be the medical director or a qualified member of the medical staff). **Stamped signatures or signing by non-physician staff are unacceptable**. In unusual circumstances, when the interpreting physician is not available, another qualified member of the medical staff may sign for them, if they choose to take such responsibility.*

> *B6.1.5 The final signed report must be transmitted to the referring health care provider within 4 working days.*

DATE: _____

Accepted by: _____ (Initials) Date_____   .

NOTES

NUCLEAR MEDICINE
B6.1.2 Interpretative Report Review Meeting
MINUTES

DATE: _____

TOPIC I

B6.1.3 An interpretation (initial or final) must be available within two (2) working days of the examination. An initial interpretation may be in the form of paper, digital storage or accessible voice system.

_____

_____

TOPIC II

B6.1.4 The final report must be reviewed and signed manually or electronically (with password protection) by the interpreting physician (who must be the medical director or a qualified member of the medical staff). Stamped signatures or signing by non-physician staff is unacceptable. In unusual circumstances, when the interpreting physician is not available, another qualified member of the medical staff may sign for them, if they choose to take such responsibility.

_____

_____

TOPIC III

B6.1.5 The final signed report must be transmitted to the referring health care provider within 4 working days

_____

_____

Medical Director or designee has reviewed the *Final Report Log* and guidelines were reviewed and discussed. The following course of action has been implemented.

_____

_____

_____   _____
Medical Director   *Date*

Medical Director or designee has reviewed the *Final Report Log* and has found no deficiencies.

_____   _____
Medical Director   *Date*

Copy: Nuclear Medicine Technologist

Accepted by: _____ (Initials) Date_____

INSERT FACILITY REPORT TEMPLATE

NOTES

INSERT FACILITY RECORD-KEEPING TEMPLATE

NUCLEAR MEDICINE
B6.1.6.5   Remote interpretations - Patient Health Information

PROCEDURE:

FAXING.
1. The Privacy and Security Rules do not prohibit faxing PHI, but you should use safeguards to ensure confidentiality.
2. Safeguards: Verify the fax numbers annually and/or pre-program common fax numbers; use a fax cover sheet with confidentiality statements (*B5.5 HIPAA FAX COVER*)

E-MAIL:
1. The Privacy and Security Rules do not prohibit the use of electronic mail to transmit PHI, as long as reasonable safeguards are used.
2. Safeguards:
   2.1.   Implement a patient "Consent for E-Mail"; verify e-mail addresses of recipients; de-identify patient information; transmit the minimum necessary; encrypt and decrypt E-PHI that you transmit.
   2.2.   drug/alcohol abuse, HIV, cancers

Do not e-mail sensitive information or diagnosis, e.g., mental health,

NUCLEAR MEDICINE
B6.1.7 Retention of Records Protocols

POLICY:
Retention of records should adhere to all state and federal regulations.
Guideline for minimum standards:

1. It is the responsibility of each facility to have knowledge of and maintain records in compliance with their own state laws.
2. Retention of records - all patient records must be confidentially maintained and be retained and accessible for minimum of three years or in compliance with state and federal law.
3. Facility will initiate a document retention policy when first indication of possible legal action.
4. Any retained hard copy will be of high quality and reflect the findings described in the final interpretation.
5. All raw digital date must be retained for a minimum of 3 years for comparison to follow-up exams or in compliance with state and federal law.
6. Technical data (such as EKG tracings) not part of the final report will be maintained as part of the facility records.
7. Worksheets for non-imaging studies are maintained as part of the facility records.

PART C   QUALITY IMPROVEMENT
SECTION C1.   QUALITY IMPROVEMENT PROGRAM
C1.1   General Quality Assessment Policies

PROCEDURE:

QUALITY ASSURANCE PLAN

Employees must attend Quality Assessment meetings

Semi-annually all personnel involved in nuclear testing must be included in the regular QA meetings. Topics will include safety procedures, improvements to be made based on quality assessments, and other information gathered throughout the period.

GOALS :
1. To make systematic and comprehensive improvements in the care of patients and nuclear cardiology services.
2. To enhance the quality of practice of the lab's health care professionals.
3. To enhance patient and staff satisfaction with services provided.

ORGANIZATION:
1. Opportunities for improvement will be identified by ongoing monitors of various aspects of care and dimensions of performance. .
2. Indicators of quality will be developed and used as a guide for the data collection and evaluation phases of the process.
3. Appropriate thresholds will be established. .
4. Action plans for corrective action will be implemented, monitored, and evaluated.
5. Communication of outcomes will be directed to appropriate individuals.

DESIGN:
1. The goal to improve will include but not be limited to: efficiency of delivery of
2. services, patient and staff safety, report generation times, image quality, patient
3. outcomes and others as appropriate

MEASURE:
1. Data collection will vary as opportunities to improve are identified. Patient surveys, incident reports, chart/report reviews, outcome studies and others will be used as appropriate.

ASSESS:
1. Data will be analyzed and evaluated based on the established indicators.
2. When thresholds have been exceeded, action plans will be implemented.

IMPROVE:
1. The improvement plan will be implemented.
2. There will be continued measurement and data analysis.

NOTES

PATIENT SURVEY

C2.1.1 Patient Satisfaction Survey

Date of exam _____ **PLEASE CIRCLE ONE**	
Were you able to locate the department easily?	YES NO
Did your referring physician explain the exam to you?	YES NO
While you were in the department, was the examination explained to your satisfaction?	YES NO
If there was a delay in starting your exam, was the reason explained to you adequately prior to your exam?	YES NO
Please rate the ease and timeliness of appointment scheduling.	Excellent Good Unsatisfactory N/A
Which word best describes the service you received from Diagnostic Imaging staff?	Excellent Good Unsatisfactory N/A
Which word best describes the service you received from Diagnostic Imaging staff?	Excellent Good Unsatisfactory N/A
Receptionist/Scheduling	Excellent Good Unsatisfactory N/A
Technologist/Nurse Excellent	Excellent Good Unsatisfactory N/A
Physician	Excellent Good Unsatisfactory N/A
Which term best describes the cleanliness of the Department	Excellent Good Unsatisfactory N/A
If you were not taken for your exam at your appointment time, how long was your wait?	
15 min 30 min. Longer than 30 minutes How long_____	

The Diagnostic Imaging staff is committed to continually improving the services we provide to all patients. We invite you to use the space on the back of this survey to give us suggestions on how we can improve our service. Your comments are most valuable, and we appreciate your time. If you prefer not to provide your name, you contribution is still appreciated.

_____
Signed   Date

Accepted by: _____ (Initials) Date_____

NOTES

PHYSICIAN SURVEY

C2.1.1 Physician Satisfaction Survey.

To improve our Imaging Services program, please complete this brief questionnaire regarding services. Your responses will assist us in providing quality care to your patients and facilitate our reporting to you. Thank you, in advance, for your time and candor in providing this information.

PLEASE RATE THE NUCLEAR CARDIOLOGY LABORATORY USING THE FOLLOWING SCALE:
1 = Excellent   2 = Very Good 3 = Good   4 = Fair   5 = Poor

_____ Departmental personnel are courteous and helpful to patients

_____ Physicians are courteous and helpful to patients

_____ Timeliness of written communications/reports to your office

_____ Timeliness of oral communication on abnormal stress exams

_____ Overall satisfaction with the clinical skills/knowledge of our departmental staff

_____ Overall satisfaction with ease of scheduling studies

_____ Overall satisfaction with the test results generated by the stress lab

_____ Overall satisfaction with the quality of care provided

_____ Confidence in recommending this lab to family/friends

_____ Overall perception to our commitment to quality

Comments: _____

_____

_____

The Diagnostic Imaging staff is committed to continually improving the services we provide to all patients. We invite you to use the space on the back of this survey to give us suggestions on how we can improve our service. Your comments are most valuable, and we appreciate your time. If you prefer not to provide your name, you contribution is still appreciated.

_____

Signed   Date

PLEASE FOLD AND LEAVE AT THE FRONT DESK.

Accepted by: _____ (Initials) Date_____   .

NOTES

NUCLEAR MEDICINE
C2.1.1 Referring Physician Satisfaction Survey

PLEASE RATE 1 = very dissatisfied, 2 = dissatisfied, 3 = neutral, 4 = satisfied, 5 = very satisfied	
CLERICAL SERVICES:	
Courtesy and helpfulness of office staff	1 2 3 4 5
Calling to make an appointment	1 2 3 4 5
Phones answered promptly & hold time is minimal	1 2 3 4 5
Timely response to voice mail messages	1 2 3 4 5
Level of knowledge/courtesy of our front desk employees	1 2 3 4 5
Front desk interaction with your patients	1 2 3 4 5
Accuracy of reports	1 2 3 4 5
Receive faxed reports when requested	1 2 3 4 5
Efficiency of film delivery	1 2 3 4 5
Courtesy of film delivery courier	1 2 3 4 5
TECHNICAL SERVICES:	1 2 3 4 5
Level of professionalism/knowledge of technical staff	1 2 3 4 5
Technologist interaction with your patients	1 2 3 4 5
Feedback from patients about technologists	1 2 3 4 5
Quality of images:	1 2 3 4 5
OVERALL SERVICES	1 2 3 4 5
Selection of appointment times	1 2 3 4 5
Availability of urgent appointments	1 2 3 4 5
Patient wait time	1 2 3 4 5
Level of knowledge/courtesy of billing office staff	1 2 3 4 5
Feedback from your patients about office staff	1 2 3 4 5
Quality of professional readings:	1 2 3 4 5
Overall experience	1 2 3 4 5
NEEDS ASSESSMENT	1 2 3 4 5
PLEASE RATE 1 not important, 2 slightly important, 3 important, 4 very important, 5 essential	
Reputation of faculty	1 2 3 4 5
Accessibility	1 2 3 4 5
Quality of diagnostic equipment	1 2 3 4 5
Travel distance for patient	1 2 3 4 5
Availability of parking	1 2 3 4 5
Participation with managed care plan	1 2 3 4 5
Availability of urgent and same-day appointments	1 2 3 4 5
Access to electronic (digital) images	1 2 3 4 5
Your Medical Specialty	
How can our services be improved?	

The Diagnostic Imaging staff is committed to continually improving the services we provide to all patients. We invite you to use the space on the back of this survey to give us suggestions on how we can improve our service. Your comments are most valuable, and we appreciate your time. If you prefer not to provide your name, you contribution is still appreciated. to us.
Name (Optional): _____ *Phone:* _____

NOTES

NUCLEAR MEDICINE
SECTION C1.   QUALITY IMPROVEMENT PROGRAM
C2.1.2   Technical Quality Assessment

PROCEDURE:

Quarterly

1. Technical Director will randomly select and review five or more patient studies
2. Complete patient information for
    C2.1.2 Technical Quality Assessment Form
    C2.1.2 Image Quality Assessment
3. Technical Director will review for 20% differential
4. Results with greater than 20% variance should be submitted to Medical Director for corrective action and discussion with technologist
5. Keep completed forms in *Technical Quality Assessment* folder

NOTES

NUCLEAR MEDICINE
C2.1.2   Technical Quality Assessment

PROCEDURE:
To assess and improve the technical quality of the images and procedures

DATE _____

NAME _____

NUCLEAR MEDICINE # _____

PROCEDURE _____

READ BY_____

QUALITY (TECHNICAL)   SATISFACTORY   UNSATISFACTORY

   1.   Name/Date Legible   _____   _____
   6.   Technical parameters   _____   _____
      6.1.   Count rate/time   _____   _____
      6.2.   Orientation _____   _____
   7.   Tech's Initials   _____   _____
   8.   Quality of Imaging   _____   _____
   9.   Prescription Attached   _____   _____

SAFETY
   ∴ Dose in Guidelines   ☐   Dose higher than guidelines   ☐

PEER REVIEW
   ∴ Acceptable   ☐   Revised   ☐

APPROPRIATENESS
   1.   According to Criteria*☐ Other   ☐
   2.   Canceled   ☐   Reason _____
   3.   Correct Diagnosis   ☐   Erroneous Diagnosis   ☐
   4.   Progress Notes ☐   Discharge Notes   ☐

CONCLUSION:
_____
_____

RECOMENDATIONS: _____
_____
_____

ACTIONS TAKEN: _____
_____
_____

NUCLEAR MEDICINE
    C2.1.2   Image Quality Assessment

PURPOSE:
    Access and improve the technical quality of the images and procedures.

DATE:_____

INDICATOR	THRESHOLD	CORRECTIVE ACTION
Camera Quality Control	☐ Varying Factors ☐ Values Met ☐ Unacceptable	Service Required
Ongoing Evaluation Of Product Performance	☐ Varying Factors ☐ Values Met ☐ Unacceptable	
Image Quality	☐ Varying Factors ☐ Indications Met ☐ Unacceptable	
Image Reproducibility	☐ Varying Factors ☐ Values Met ☐ Unacceptable	
Quantitative Results	☐ Varying Factors ☐ Values Met ☐ Unacceptable	
Medical Events	☐ Varying Factors ☐ Indications Met ☐ Unacceptable	
Radioactive Spills	☐ Varying Factors ☐ Indications Met ☐ Unacceptable	
Adverse Effects	☐ Varying Factors ☐ Within Limits ☐ Unacceptable	
Images Display	☐ Indications Met ☐ Within Limits ☐ Unacceptable	
Comparison Testing [Phantom Program]	☐ Indications Met ☐ Within Limits ☐ Unacceptable	

Accepted by: _____ (Initials) Date_____   .

NUCLEAR MEDICINE

C2.1.3   Interpretive Quality Assessment
Physician Technical Quality Assessment

PROCEDURE:

1. Nuclear Technologist will create a "Quality Assurance" for each Physician that will conduct peer review.
2. Nuclear Technologist will randomly select each quarter of the year fifteen (15) or more (patient) films
3. Attached to patient records a printed and filled-in copy of
   C2.1.3   Catheterization Correlation Form
4. Place in folder of physician other than original interpreting physician

OR

If facility only generates computer patient records and physician will read on computer submit in folder for each patient just printed and filled-in copy of form C2.1.3 Catheterization Correlation Form

5. Quarterly submit forms to "Quality Assurance Physician Name" folder to selected physician.
6. Keep Physician's completed forms in in "Quality Assessment" folder
7. Conduct annual review for 20% differential
8. If greater than 20% disagreement, submit record to Medical Director for corrective action and discussion with reading physician

NUCLEAR MEDICINE

C2.1.3 Catheterization Correlation Forms

PURPOSE:

Interpretive Quality Assessment
Quality Assurance Activity Report

PROCEDURE:

Data collection timeframe: from_____ to_____

Indicator: Correlation of Nuclear Findings with Cardiac Catheterization *Threshold:* 80% correlation

Corrective Action: When threshold is exceeded; cases are reviewed by the interpreting physicians and discrepancies are discussed.

Patient	Scan Date	Nuclear Results	Cath Date	Cath Results	Correlate	Reviews(Results)
					Yes No	
					Yes No	
					Yes No	
					Yes No	
					Yes No	

Review of correlation data:
- ☐ The nuclear findings and Cath reports correlated within the 80% threshold.
- ☐ The nuclear findings and Cath reports did not correlate within the 80% threshold.
- ☐ The nuclear cases were reviewed and the discrepancies can be explained by:
- ☐ Breast attenuation
- ☐ Technical difficulties (pt motion, body habitus)
- ☐ Non-diagnostic stress test
- ☐ Processing technique
- ☐ Interpretation (overread) other:_____
- ☐ Findings were discussed with appropriate staff.
- ☐ Suggested follow-up:_____

_____
Reviewing Physician

Accepted by: _____ (Initials) Date_____ .

MINUTES

C3.2	**Semi-Annual Quality Assessment Meeting Minutes**

ATTACH FORMS

C3.   Quality Assessment Report

C3.2   Semi-Annual Quality Assessment Report

Date: _____

TOPIC I *(Previous Business)*

_____

_____

_____

_____

_____

_____

_____

_____

_____

TOPIC II
(New Business)

_____

_____

_____

_____

_____

_____

_____

_____

ATTENDED BY:

_____

_____

_____

_____

_____

_____

Recorded by: _____ (Initials) Date_____   .

NOTES

NUCLEAR MEDICINE

C3.2   Quality Assessment Report

DATE:_____

INDICATOR	THRESHOLD	CORRECTIVE ACTION
Appropriateness of procedures	☐ Varying Factors ☐ Indications Met ☐ Unacceptable	
Written Orders	☐ Varying Factors ☐ Indications Met ☐ Unacceptable	
Scheduling backlogs	☐ Varying Factors ☐ Indications Met ☐ Unacceptable	
Late reports	☐ Varying Factors ☐ Indications Met ☐ Unacceptable	
Patient wait times	☐ Varying Factors ☐ Within Limits ☐ Unacceptable	
Special Needs Patients Met	☐ Varying Factors ☐ Within Limits ☐ Unacceptable	
	☐ Varying Factors ☐ Within Limits ☐ Unacceptable	
	☐ Varying Factors ☐ Within Limits ☐ Unacceptable	

Accepted by: _____ *(Initials) Date*_____   .

NOTES

NUCLEAR MEDICINE
SECTION C3.   QUALITY ASSESSMENT REPORT
C3.2   Semi-Annual Quality Assessment meetings
QUALITY ASSESSMENT REPORT   DATE_____

INDICATORS	THRESHOLD	CORRECTIVE ACTION
CATH CORRELATION	80% Correlation	Case Reviews Technical Factors Assessed
PATIENT OUTCOME		Case Reviews Technical Factors Assessed
CAMERA QC	Within Manufacturer's Spec's	Recalibration Service Upgrades Considered
RADIATION SAFETY	100% Compliance	RSO Review
IMAGE QUALITY	100% Diagnostic Quality	Study Repeated Artifacts Identified And Corrected
REPORT TURNAROUND	100% Within 48 Hrs	Work Flow Resource Utilization Improvements New Technologies Implemented
PATIENT SATISFACTION	80% Within Benchmarks Of Good To Excellent	Areas Of Improvement Discussed Implemented Re-Survey
PATIENT SAFETY	Doses Within 10%	Calibration Times Reviewed Late Patients Reviewed Improvements
REPRODUCIBILITY	80% Correlation Between Interpreting Physicians	Case Reviews
PHYSICIAN SATISFACTION	80% Within Benchmarks Of Good To Excellent	Areas Of Improvement Implemented Re-Survey
DISCUSS FEEDBACK AT NEXT QA MEETING		
NEGATIVE RESPONSES ADDRESSED BY THE APPROPRIATE PERSONNEL WITHIN 30 DAYS		
CORRECTIVE ACTION		
FOLLOW-UP NEEDED:		

☐   Results will be evaluated. (6-12 months) The improvement(s) will be instituted.

☐   Corrective action will be monitored for its effectiveness by looking at these indicators 6-12 months later and evaluating if the improvement has successfully been implemented.

☐   Quality assurance activities will be discussed at regularly scheduled staff meetings.

☐   The agenda and attendance will be documented.

Accepted by: _____ (Initials) Date_____

NOTES

DIRECTORY OF ILLUSTRATIONS

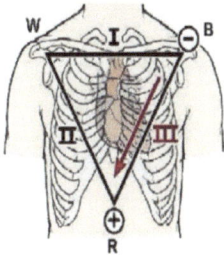

B2.3 12-ACC AHA Lead Placement

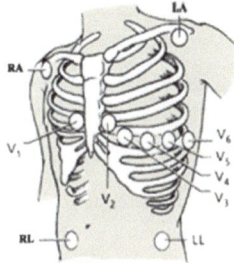

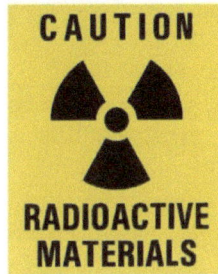

B2.3 12-ACC AHA Lead Placement

B4.3.1.2 Radioactive Materials Signage

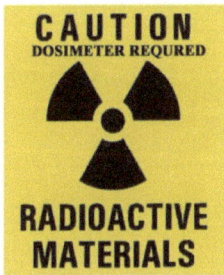

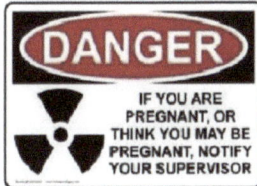

B4.3.1.2 Radioactive Materials Signage

B4.3.1.4 Employee Radiation Safety

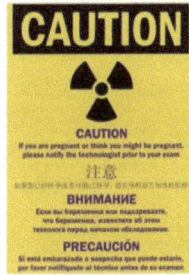

B4.3.1.4 Employee Radiation Safety

B4.3.1.9 Radioactive Spill Policy

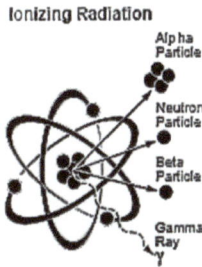

B4.3.1.9 Spill Ionizing Radiation

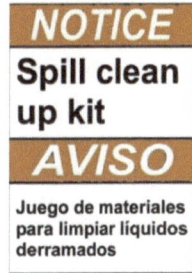

B4.3.1.9 Spill Kit

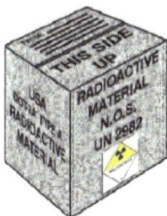

B4.3.2 Survey of Radioactive Shipments

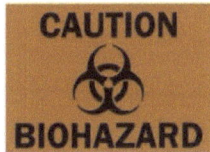

B5.8 Infection Control

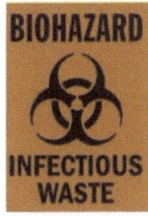

B5.8 Infection Control Waste

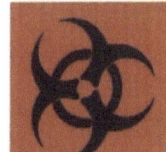

OSHA FACT SHEET

	DIRECTORY OF PRINTABLE FORMS AVAILABLE ON PURCHASED CD**
1.	A Structure Organization
2.	A1 Memo Review PP Manual
3.	A4.2 Equipment and Instrumentation in Use
4.	B1.1.4 Employee Orientation-Annual
5.	B2.1 Facility Clinical Procedure Protocols
6.	B2.1.1 Patient Identification
7.	B2.1.2.3 Fetal Exposure
8.	B2.1.4 Pregnancy and Breastfeeding Questionnaire
9.	B2.1.3 Pregnancy and Breastfeeding Instruction
10.	B2.2 Diagnostic Imaging Procedure Protocol
11.	B2.2 Dobutamine Dose Infusion Chart
12.	B2.2 Dobutamine Stress Flow Sheet
13.	B2.2 Adenosine Cardiolite Stress Chart
14.	B2.2 Myocardial Perfusion Imaging Same-Day Rest-Stress Tc99m
15.	B2.2 Myocardial Perfusion Imaging Same-Day Rest Stress Tc99m Myoview Phillips EXAMPLE ONLY
16.	B2.2 MPI 1-Day Rest Stress Gated GE Ventri EXAMPLE ONLY
17.	B2.2 Rest Equilibrium Nuclear Angiography (Rest MUGA) EXAMPLE ONLY
18.	B2.2 Myoview Dobutamine Infusion Protocol
19.	B2.2 Myoview Screening Questionnaire
20.	B2.3 Adenosine Cardiolite (Sestamibi)GE Ventri EXAMPLE ONLY
21.	B2.3 MPI Exercise Stress with Bruce Protocol
22.	B2.3 -Six Minute Adenosine Stress Protocol
23.	B2.2 Cardiolite Treadmill EKG Chart
24.	B2.3 Bruce Modified Low Chart
25.	B2.4.2 Patient Instructions
26.	B3.2 Imaging Equipment Quality Control Log
27.	B3.3.2 Medical Emergencies Crash Cart Review
28.	B4 Annual Radiation Safety Officer Review
29.	B4. Radiation Safety Officer Meeting Minutes
30.	B4.1.2 Delegation of Authority MEMO
31.	B4.1.3 Delegation of Who May Handle RAM
32.	B4.1.3 Authorization of NMT to Handle RAM
33.	B4.1.3 Designation Who May Handle RAM
34.	B4.3.1.11 Record Of Dose Rate And Contamination Survey
35.	B4.3.1.15 Nuclear Pharmacy Card
36.	B4.3.1.15 Instructions for Family of Released Radiation Patients
37.	B4.3.1.3 Daily Spot Checks for RAM Contamination Chart
38.	B4.3.1.4 Employee RAM Orientation-Annual Checklist
39.	B4.3.1.4 Housekeeping Radiation Safety Training
40.	B4.3.1.5 Missing Dosimeter
41.	B4.3.1.5 Radiation Dosimetry Report
42.	B4.3.1.6 Declaration of Pregnancy for Personnel
43.	B4.3.1.6 Receipt of Declaration Of Pregnancy
44.	B4.3.1.9 Radioactive Spill Form

		DIRECTORY OF PRINTABLE FORMS AVAILABLE ON PURCHASED CD**
		B4.3.1.9 Spill Procedure Sign
45.		B4.3.2 Receipt of RAM MEMO
46.		B5. HIPAA FAX Cover
47.		B5.1.5 Incident Occurrence Report
48.		B5.11 Code Plan of Action
49.		B5.2 Written Requests for Services
50.		B5.3 Duties Responsibilities of Staff
51.		B5.4 Safety Security for Staff and Patients
52.		B5.5 Employee HIPAA Confidentiality
53.		B5.5 HIPAA Consent To The Use And Disclosure
54.		B5.6 Consent for Nuclear Cardiology
55.		B5.6 Informed Consent
56.		B6.1.2 Interpretative Report Review Meeting
57.		B6.1.2 Interpretive Report Timeliness Requirements
58.		B6.1.2 Reports Meeting Minutes
59.		C2.1.1 Patient Satisfaction Survey
60.		C2.1.1 Physician Satisfaction Survey
61.		C2.1.1 Referring Physician Survey
62.		C2.1.2 Image Quality Assessment
63.		C2.1.2 Technical Quality Assessment
64.		C2.1.3 Catheterization Correlation
65.		C3.2 Semi-Annual Quality Assessment Meeting Minutes
66.		C3. Quality Assessment Report
67.		C3.2 Semi-Annual Quality Assessment Report

SITES OF INTEREST
RESOURCES:

1. American College of Cardiology
   http://www.cardiosource.org/

2. Society of Nuclear Medicine and Molecular Imaging
   http://www.snmmi.org/

3. Louisiana Department of Environmental Quality DEQ
   http://www.deq.louisiana.gov/

4. HIPAA - General Information
   http://www.cms.gov/

5. U.S. Nuclear Regulatory Commission
   http://www.regulations.gov/

9. Centers for Medicare & Medicaid Services
   http://www.cms.gov/

10. Hazardous Materials Safety Administration (PHMSA)
    phmsa.dot.gov/hazmat

6. *Intersocietal Accreditation Commission*
   IAC Policies & Procedures
   http://www.intersocietal.org/intersocietal.htm

7. American Heart Association
   http://www.heart.org/HEARTORG/

11. National Center for Missing and Exploited Children
    http://www.missingkids.com/home

www.ingramcontent.com/pod-product-compliance
Lightning Source LLC
Chambersburg PA
CBHW041725210326
41598CB00008B/780